CW01176023

THE COMPLETE ANTI-INFLAMMATORY DIET FOR BEGINNERS

Easy Recipes to Improve your Immune System and Restore Overall Health

Copyright © 2021
Gina Dasy Wertmullen
All rights reserved

This document is geared towards providing exact and reliable information in regards to the topic and issue covered. The publication is sold with the idea that the publisher is not required to render accounting, officially permitted, or otherwise, qualified services. If advice is necessary, legal or professional, a practiced individual in the profession should be ordered. From a Declaration of Principles which was accepted and approved equally by a Committee of the American bar association and a Committee of Publishersand Associations.In no way is it legal to reproduce, duplicate, or transmit any part of this document in either electronic means or in printed format. Recording of this publication is strictly prohibited and any storage of this document is not allowed unless with written permission from the publisher. All rights reserved. The information provided herein is stated to be truthful and consistent, in that any liability, in terms of inattention or otherwise, by any usage or abuse of any policies, processes, or directions contained within is the solitary and user responsibility of the recipient reader. Under no circumstances will any legal responsibility or blame be held against the publisher for any reparation, damages, or monetary loss due to the information herein, either directly or indirectly. Respective authors own all copyrights not held by the publisher. The information herein is offered for informational purposes solely and is universal as so. The presentation of the information is without contract or any type of guarantee assurance. The trademarks that are used are without any consent, and the publication of the trademark is without permission or backing by the trademark owner. All trademarks and brands within this book are for clarifying purposes only and are the owned by the owners themselves, not affiliated with this document. The material in this book is for informational purposes only. As each individual situation is unique, you should use proper discretion, in consultation with healthcare practitioner, before undertaking the protocols, diet, exercises, techniques, training methods, or otherwise described herein. The author and publisher expressly disclaim responsibility for any adverse effects that may result fromtheuseor application of the information contained herein.

Recipes

7	INTRODUCTION
10	Crusted Salmon
11	Tuna-Spinach Salad
12	Matcha Green Tea Latte
13	Roasted Salmon with Cranberry Relish
14	Lentil Soup
15	Spiced Pecans
16	Berry-Almond Smoothie
17	Roasted Salmon with Chickpeas & Greens
18	Herbal Chamomile Health Tonic
19	Miso-Maple Salmon
20	Cauliflower & Broccoli Salad
21	Garlic Roasted Salmon & Brussels Sprouts
22	Carrot Cake Energy Bites
23	Almond-Matcha Green Smoothie
24	Easy Saag Paneer
25	Spinach Salad with Roasted Sweet Potatoes, White Beans & Basil
26	Salmon & Fall Vegetables

27	Green Salad with Edamame & Beets
28	Roasted Beet Hummus
29	Peach, Raspberry & Watercress Salad with Five-Spice Bacon
30	Turmeric Latte
31	Purple Fruit Salad
32	Beet & Goat Cheese Tartines
33	Spinach Salad
34	Turmeric-Ginger Tahini Dip
35	Miso Soup Cup of Noodles with Shrimp & Green Tea Soba
36	Romaine Wedges with Sardines & Caramelized Onions
37	Orange, Anchovy & Olive Salad
38	Spinach-Avocado Smoothie
39	Roasted Root Veggies & Greens over Spiced Lentils
40	Tangerine & Roasted Beet Salad with Feta & Pistachios
41	Green Tea-Peach Smoothie
42	Cranberry-Almond Granola Bars
43	Blueberry Almond Chia Pudding
44	Citrus Salad with Ginger Yogurt
45	Red Bell Pepper, Spinach, and Goat Cheese Salad
46	Roasted Root Vegetables
47	Brussels Sprouts and Carrots
48	Chilled Red Bell Pepper and Habanero Soup
49	Foil Packet Potatoes and Eggs
50	Curried Chicken Salad with Spiced Chickpeas and Raita

51   Oat Porridge with Fruit

52   Dukkah Roasted

53   Chickpea and Vegetable Coconut Curry

54   Zucchini Taco

55   Marinated Tomatoes and Mushrooms

56   Eggplant Caponata

57   Indian Freezer Appetizer

58   Artichoke Ricotta Flatbread

59   Lemon Chicken with Asparagus

60   Garlic Shrimp

61   Greek Chicken With Tomato, Olive, And Feta Topping

62   Green Curry

63   Roasted Fish with Vegetables

64   Chicken Quinoa Fried Rice

65   Lemon Chicken & Potatoes with Kale

66   Chicken Kebabs with Mediterranean Couscous

67   Greek Kale Salad with Quinoa & Chicken

68   Vegan Coconut Chickpea Curry

69   Sheet-Pan Chicken Fajita

70   Cauliflower with Chickpeas

71   Plaice with Thai Coconut Curry Sauce

72   Slow-Cooker Southwest Quinoa

73   Italian Soup

74   Chicken & Farro Herb Salad

75	Sheet-Pan Chicken & Vegetables
76	Baked Salmon & Vegetables
77	Easy Anti-inflammatory Water
78	Lemon Chicken Orzo Soup
79	Charred Shrimp & Pesto
80	Turkey Meatballs with Linguine & Fresh Tomato Sauce
81	Chicken, Arugula & Butternut Squash Salad with Brussels Sprouts
82	Roasted Salmon with Smoky Chickpeas & Greens
83	Jackfruit Barbacoa Burrito
84	Chicken, Quinoa & Sweet Potato Casserole
85	Moroccan Baked Cod & Vegetables with Chermoula Sauce
86	Ratatouille
87	Roasted Cauliflower
88	Salmon Salad
89	Smoked Salmon
90	Eggplant Pizza Bites with Spinach and Mushrooms
91	Lemon Roasted Broccoli
92	Speedy Salmon Patties
93	Minestrone
94	Oven Roasted Tomatoes
95	Florence White Bean Soup
96	Zucchini with Egg
97	Creamy White Bean Soup

INTRODUCTION

It is said that health is achieved first of all at the table, by eating foods that have beneficial properties for the body.

A useful diet to combat premature aging and many other ailments is the anti-inflammatory diet.

Inflammation is a series of processes by which the body reacts to the action of harmful agents, such as bacteria or viruses, or to the external or internal damage it may encounter.

Normally, inflammation resolves naturally after a few days, but, in some cases, it can become chronic, giving rise to periods of pain of varying intensity and duration.

Gastritis or arthritis are the most common manifestations of chronic inflammation.

Proper nutrition, combined with effective therapy, can restore good health.

Some foods have very strong anti-inflammatory properties, while other foods should be avoided.

It is also important to evaluate the amount of energy our body needs through food intake.

The elements of the anti-inflammatory diet:

The initial phase of the anti-inflammatory diet is to reduce the calories we eat in our food.

Reducing calories consumed promotes the reduction of inflammation.

To reduce calories, it is not strictly necessary to eat little and badly, but to reduce calorie consumption by 25/30% based on gender and age and to vary the ingredients of the diet.

Calorie reduction:
- lowers cholesterol and triglyceride levels
- increases HDL (good cholesterol)
- extends the life of cells
- reduces inflammation
- fights oxidative stress
- counteracts neuro-degenerative diseases
- slows down skin aging
- when combined with regular physical activity, increases life expectancy by 5-10 years.

Some foods with anti-inflammatory properties are:
- cereals
- whole foods
- fruits and vegetables (e.g. spinach, cabbage, strawberries, blueberries, cherries, oranges)
- fatty fish such as salmon, mackerel, tuna and sardines
- spices: turmeric and ginger are great

- tomatoes

- olive oil.

Foods to avoid:

- all types of fats

- refined carbohydrates, such as white bread and pastries

- fefined flours

- sugars

- dairy products and sausages

- red meat (burgers, steaks)

- processed meat (hot dog, sausage)

- French fries and other fried foods

- sweetened drinks.

Always remember that a healthy diet is useful not only for reducing the risk of chronic diseases, but also for improving mood and overall quality of life.

Below you will find a series of recipes to be included in your diet. Once you have replaced the meals with those in this book, I suggest you check your new daily calorie intake, and reduce it by 20/30%.

For a perfect reduction in calorie intake, a consultation with a dietician is recommended.

Crusted Salmon

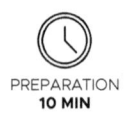

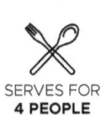

FISH

PREPARATION
10 MIN

SERVES FOR
4 PEOPLE

INGREDIENTS

1/2 teaspoon honey
1/2 teaspoon kosher salt
1/4 teaspoon lemon zest
1/4 teaspoon crushed red pepper
1 teaspoon lemon juice
1 teaspoon chopped fresh rosemary
1 clove garlic, minced
1 teaspoon extra-virgin olive oil
1 skinless salmon fillet, fresh
2 teaspoons Dijon mustard
3 tablespoons panko breadcrumbs
3 tablespoons finely chopped walnuts
Chopped fresh parsley and lemon wedges for garnish
Olive oil cooking spray

STEPS

1. Preheat oven to 425 degrees F. Line a rimmed baking sheet with parchment paper.
2. Add lemon juice, mustard, garlic, lemon zest, honey, rosemary, salt and crushed red pepper in a bowl. In other bowl combine walnuts, panko and oil.
3. Transfer salmon on the prepared baking sheet. Spread the mustard mixture over the fish and sprinkle with the panko mixture.
4. Bake for about 10 minutes.
5. Add parsley and serve with lemon wedges.

NUTRITION FACTS

Per Serving:
222 calories
protein 24g
carbohydrates 4g
fat 12g
saturated fat 2g
cholesterol 62mg
sodium 256mg
sugars 1g

Tuna-Spinach Salad

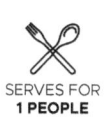

FISH

PREPARATION
5 MIN

SERVES FOR
1 PEOPLE

INGREDIENTS

1 medium orange, peeled or sliced
1 5-ounce can chunk light tuna in water, drained
1 1/2 tablespoons tahini
1 1/2 tablespoons lemon juice
1 1/2 tablespoons water
2 tablespoons feta cheese
2 tablespoons parsley
2 cups baby spinach
4 Kalamata olives, pitted and chopped

STEPS

1. In a bowl add, lemon juice, water, tahini and whisk together. Add parsley, olives, feta, and tuna; stir to combine. Serve the tuna salad over 2 cups of spinach and orange.

NUTRITION FACTS

Per Serving:
376 calories
protein 25.7g
carbohydrates 26.2g
fat 21g
saturated fat 5.2g
cholesterol 46.3mg
sodium 664.8mg
fiber 5.8g
sugars 13.9g

Matcha Green Tea Latte

BEVERAGE

PREPARATION
10 MIN

SERVES FOR
1 PEOPLE

INGREDIENTS

1/2 cup boiling water
1 cup low-fat milk
1 teaspoon honey
1 teaspoon matcha tea powder

STEPS

1. Blend boiling water with matcha powder in a blender until foamy. Heat milk with honey. Whisk the milk until frothy. Pour the milk into a mug, then add in the tea.

NUTRITION FACTS

Per Serving:

124 calories
protein 8.2g
carbohydrates 17.9g
fat 2.4g
saturated fat 1.5g
cholesterol 12.2mg
sodium 109.4mg
sugars 17.9g

Roasted Salmon with Cranberry Relish

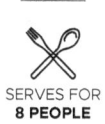

FISH

PREPARATION
30 MIN

SERVES FOR
8 PEOPLE

INGREDIENTS

1/2 teaspoon whole black peppercorns, cracked
1 small shallot, minced
1 serrano pepper, seeded
1 medium Granny Smith apple, peeled and finely diced
1 stalk celery, finely diced
1 lemon, zested and cut into wedges
1 tablespoon balsamic vinegar
1 1/2 teaspoons kosher salt, divided
2 1/2 pounds skin-on salmon fillet
2 cloves garlic, peeled and chopped
2 tablespoons extra-virgin olive oil, divided
2 teaspoons Dijon mustard
2 tablespoons chopped fresh parsley, divided
8 ounces frersh cranberries

STEPS

1. Line a rimmed baking sheet with parchment paper.
2. Preheat oven to 425 degrees F.
3. Transfer the salmon to the prepared pan. Mash garlic, lemon zest, peppercorns, and 1 teaspoon salt, into a paste with a fork. Place to a bowl and add 1 tablespoon oil and mustard. Spread on the salmon. Bake for about 13 minutes.
4. Place cranberries, shallot, and serrano in a food processor until finely chopped. Transfer to a bowl in apple, 1/2 teaspoon salt, 1 tablespoon parsley and celery, vinegar, and the remaining 1 tablespoon oil.
5. Sprinkle the salmon with 1 tablespoon parsley and serve with the relish and lemon wedges.

NUTRITION FACTS

Serving Size: About 1 1/4 Cups
Per Serving:

229 calories
protein 28.6g
carbohydrates 7.6g
fat 8.8g
cholesterol 66.3mg
sodium 452.4mg
fiber 1.7g
sugars 4g

Lentil Soup

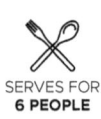

SOUP

PREPARATION
10 MIN

SERVES FOR
6 PEOPLE

INGREDIENTS

3/4 teaspoon salt
1/4 cup packed fresh flat-leaf parsley leaves
1 cup chopped yellow onion
1 cup chopped carrots
1 cup chopped turnip
1 tablespoon chopped fresh thyme
1 1/2 tablespoons balsamic vinegar
2 tablespoons extra-virgin olive oil, divided
2 cups brown lentils, rinsed
3 radishes, cut into matchsticks
5 cups fresh baby spinach
6 cups low-sodium vegetable broth

STEPS

1. Select Sauté setting on a programmable pressure multicooker. Select a High-temperature setting and allow it to preheat. Add 1 tablespoon oil, onion, carrots, turnip, and thyme; cook, stirring for 5 minutes. Add in broth, lentils, and salt.
2. Press Cancel. Cover the cooker and lock the lid in place. Turn the steam release handle to the Sealing position. Select Manual/Pressure Cook setting. Select High pressure for 10 minutes.
3. When cooking is complete, carefully turn the steam release handle to Venting position and let the steam fully escape before removing the lid from the cooker. Add in vinegar and spinach.
4. In a small bowl toss parsley and radishes with 1 tablespoon oil. Ladle the soup into 6 bowls and garnish with the radish mixture.
5. Serve.

NUTRITION FACTS

Per Serving:

305 calories
protein 18g
carbohydrates 47.5g
fat 5.5g
saturated fat 0.8g
sodium 470mg
fiber 17.7g
sugars 8.8g

Spiced Pecans

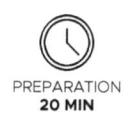

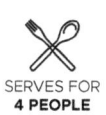

SIDE

PREPARATION
20 MIN

SERVES FOR
4 PEOPLE

INGREDIENTS

1/4 teaspoon ground allspice
1/4 teaspoon ground cloves
1/4 teaspoon ground nutmeg
1/2 teaspoon salt
1 large egg white
1 tablespoon water
1 pound pecan halves
6 tablespoons superfine sugar
Pinch of ground cinnamon
Pinch of cayenne pepper

STEPS

1. Line a rimmed baking sheet with parchment paper.
2. Preheat oven to 300 degrees F.
3. Whisk egg white, water, nutmeg, sugar, salt, allspice, cloves, cayenne, and cinnamon in a bowl. Add pecans and stir. Spread in a single layer on the prepared pan.
4. Bake for 60 minutes. Let cool for 20 minutes. Break apart before serving.

NUTRITION FACTS

Serving Size: 1/4 Cup
Per Serving:

152 calories
protein 2g
carbohydrates 6.4g
fat 14.3g
saturated fat 1.2g
sodium 50mg
fiber 1.9g
sugars 4.4g

Berry-Almond Smoothie

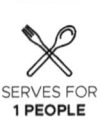

SMOOTHIE

PREPARATION
10 MIN

SERVES FOR
1 PEOPLE

INGREDIENTS

1/8 teaspoon ground cardamom
1/8 teaspoon vanilla extract
1/4 cup blueberries
1/4 teaspoon ground cinnamon
1/2 cup frozen sliced banana
1/2 cup plain unsweetened almond milk
2/3 cup frozen raspberries
1 tablespoon unsweetened coconut flakes
5 tablespoons sliced almonds, divided

STEPS

1. Blend a banana, raspberries, 3 tablespoons almonds, almond milk, cinnamon, cardamom, and vanilla in a blender until very smooth.
2. Pour the smoothie into a bowl and top with the remaining 2 tablespoons almonds blueberries, and coconut.

NUTRITION FACTS

Serving Size:1 1/3 Cups
Per Serving:

360 calories
protein 9.2g
carbohydrates 45.6g
fat 19g
saturated fat 3.3g
sodium 89.4mg
fiber 14g
sugars 21.4g

Roasted Salmon with Chickpeas & Greens

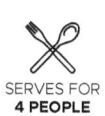

FISH

PREPARATION
40 MIN

SERVES FOR
4 PEOPLE

INGREDIENTS

1/4 cup mayonnaise
1/4 cup chopped fresh chives and/or dill, plus more for garnish
1/4 teaspoon ground pepper, divided
1/4 cup water
1/2 teaspoon salt, divided, plus a pinch
1/2 teaspoon garlic powder
1/3 cup buttermilk
1 tablespoon smoked paprika
1 1/4 pounds wild salmon, cut into 4 portions
2 tablespoons extra-virgin olive oil, divided
15 ounce can no-salt-added chickpeas, rinsed
10 cups chopped kale

NUTRITION FACTS

Per Serving:

447 calories
protein 37g
carbohydrates 23.4g
fat 21.8g
saturated fat 3.7g
sodium 556.7mg
fiber 6.4g
sugars 2.2g

STEPS

1. Preheat oven to 425 degrees F. In a bowl adds 1 tablespoon oil, paprika, and 1/4 teaspoon salt. Thoroughly pat chickpeas dry, then toss with the paprika mixture. Spread on a rimmed baking sheet. Bake the chickpeas for 30 minutes.
2. Combine, mayonnaise, 1/4 teaspoon pepper, garlic powder, puree buttermilk, and herbs, in a blender until smooth. Set aside.
3. Heat the 1 tablespoon oil in a skillet over medium heat. Add kale and cook, for 2 minutes. Add water and continue cooking 5 minutes more. Remove from heat and stir in a pinch of salt.
4. Remove the chickpeas from the oven and push them to one side of the pan. Place salmon on the other side and season with the remaining 1/4 teaspoon each salt and pepper. Bake until the salmon is just cooked through.
5. Drizzle the reserved dressing on the salmon, garnish with more herbs, and serve with kale and chickpeas.

Herbal Chamomile Health Tonic

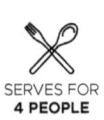

TEA

PREPARATION
5 MIN

SERVES FOR
4 PEOPLE

INGREDIENTS

2 sprigs rosemary, lightly bruised
2 teaspoons grated fresh ginger
2-4 teaspoons honey
4 cups boiling water
4 slices lemon
6 bags chamomile tea

STEPS

1. Stir boiling water, tea bags, rosemary, ginger, lemon, honey, in a heatproof bowl. Steep, stirring occasionally, for 20 minutes. Strain the liquid through a fine-mesh sieve, pressing on the tea bags to get as much liquid out as possible.

NUTRITION FACTS

Serving Size: 1 Cup
Per Serving:

6 calories
protein 0.1g
carbohydrates 1.2g
sodium 3.1mg
sugars 3g

Miso-Maple Salmon

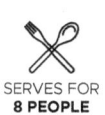

FISH

PREPARATION
15 MIN

SERVES FOR
8 PEOPLE

INGREDIENTS

1/4 teaspoon ground pepper
1/4 cup white miso
1 skin-on salmon fillet
2 lemons
2 limes
2 tablespoons extra-virgin olive oil
2 tablespoons maple syrup
Pinch of cayenne pepper
Sliced scallions for garnish

STEPS

1. Line a large rimmed baking sheet with foil.
2. Preheat oven broiler to high.
3. Juice 1 lime and 1 lemon into a bowl. Whisk in miso, oil maple syrup, pepper, and cayenne. Place salmon, skin-side down, on the prepared pan, and spread the miso mixture on top. Halve the remaining lemon and lime and arrange around the salmon.
4. Broil the salmon for 10 minutes. Serve with the lemon and lime halves and sprinkle with scallions.

NUTRITION FACTS

Serving Size: 4 Oz. Salmon
Per Serving:

230 calories
protein 28.3g
carbohydrates 6.7g
fat 8.7g
cholesterol 63.3mg
sodium 340.7mg
fiber 0.1g
sugars 3.3g

Cauliflower & Broccoli Salad

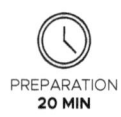

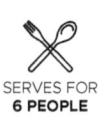

SALAD

PREPARATION
20 MIN

SERVES FOR
6 PEOPLE

INGREDIENTS

1/4 teaspoon ground pepper
1/3 cup chopped toasted pecans
1/2 teaspoon salt, divided
1/2 cup dried cherries
1 tablespoon champagne vinegar
1 teaspoon honey
1 1/2 teaspoons Dijon mustard
2 ounces shaved manchego cheese
3 cups cauliflower florets
3 cups broccoli florets
4 tablespoons extra-virgin olive oil, divided
8 cups chopped lacinato kale

STEPS

1. Preheat oven to 450 degrees F.
2. Places cauliflower and broccoli in a bowl. Add 1/4 teaspoon salt, pepper, 2 tablespoons oil, and toss. Spread on the preheated baking sheet and roast, turning once halfway through, cooking about 10 minutes. Let cool.
3. Meanwhile, whisk mustard, honey vinegar, and the remaining 2 tablespoons oil and 1/4 teaspoon salt in a bowl. Add kale and combine dressing into the leaves until they are softened for about 2 minutes. Add the roasted vegetables along with cherries, cheese, and pecans, toss to combine.

NUTRITION FACTS

Serving Size: 1 1/2 Cups
Per Serving:

259 calories
protein 8.4g
carbohydrates 23.2g
fat 16.3g
cholesterol 6.8mg
sodium 321mg
fiber 4.9g
sugars 8.3g

Garlic Roasted Salmon & Brussels Sprouts

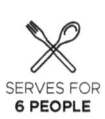

FISH

PREPARATION
45 MIN

SERVES FOR
6 PEOPLE

INGREDIENTS

3/4 cup white wine, preferably Chardonnay
3/4 teaspoon freshly ground pepper, divided
1/4 cup extra-virgin olive oil
1 teaspoon salt, divided
2 tablespoons finely chopped fresh oregano, divided
2 pounds wild-caught salmon fillet, skinned, cut into 6 portions
6 cups Brussels sprouts, trimmed and sliced
14 large cloves garlic, divided
Lemon wedges

STEPS

1. Preheat oven to 450 degrees F.
2. Mince 2 garlic cloves and combine in a bowl with oil, 1/2 teaspoon salt, 1/4 teaspoon pepper, and 1 tablespoon oregano. Halve the remaining garlic and toss with Brussels sprouts and 3 tablespoons of the seasoned oil in a roasting pan. Roast for 15 minutes.
3. Add wine to the remaining oil mixture. Remove the pan from the oven, stir the vegetables and place salmon on top. Garnish with the wine mixture. Sprinkle with the remaining 1 tablespoon salt, pepper, and 1/2 teaspoon of oregano. Bake until the salmon is just cooked through for 10 minutes. Serve with lemon wedges.

NUTRITION FACTS

Per Serving:

334 calories
protein 33g
carbohydrates 10.3g
fat 15.4g
saturated fat 2.8g
sodium 486mg
fiber 2.7g
sugars 2g

Carrot Cake Energy Bites

CAKE

PREPARATION
15 MIN

SERVES FOR
22 PORTIONS

INGREDIENTS

3/4 teaspoon ground cinnamon
1/4 cup chopped pecans
1/4 cup chia seeds
1/4 teaspoon ground turmeric
1/4 teaspoon salt
1/2 teaspoon ground ginger
1/2 cup old-fashioned rolled oats
1 cup pitted dates
1 teaspoon vanilla extract
2 medium carrots finely chopped
Pinch of ground pepper

STEPS

1. Combine chia seeds, oats, pecans, dates, in a food processor.
2. Pulse until well chopped and combined.
3. Add vanilla, cinnamon, ginger, turmeric, carrots, salt, and pepper; process until all ingredients are well chopped and a paste begins to form.
4. Roll the mixture into balls using a small Tbsp.

NUTRITION FACTS

Per Serving:

48 calories
protein 0.9g
carbohydrates 8.2g
fat 1.7g
saturated fat 0.2g
sodium 30.4mg
fiber 1.6g
sugars 5.1g

Almond-Matcha Green Smoothie

SMOOTHIE

PREPARATION
10 MIN

SERVES FOR
1 PEOPLE

INGREDIENTS

1/2 ripe kiwi, diced
1/2 cup frozen sliced banana
1/2 cup frozen sliced peaches
1/2 cup unsweetened almond milk
1 cup fresh spinach
1 teaspoon maple syrup
1 1/2 teaspoons matcha tea powder
5 tablespoons slivered almonds, divided

STEPS

1. Blend spinach, matcha, banana, peaches, almond milk, maple syrup, and 3 tablespoons almonds, in a blender until very smooth.
2. Pour the smoothie into a bowl and top with kiwi and the remaining 2 tablespoons slivered almonds.

NUTRITION FACTS

Serving Size: 1 1/2 Cups
Per Serving:

353 calories
protein 9.9g
carbohydrates 44.3g
fat 18.6g
saturated fat 1.4g
sodium 99.9mg
fiber 9.3g
sugars 25g

Easy Saag Paneer

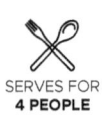

SIDE

PREPARATION
25 MIN

SERVES FOR
4 PEOPLE

INGREDIENTS

1/4 teaspoon ground turmeric
3/4 teaspoon salt
1 clove garlic, minced
1 tablespoon minced fresh ginger
1 small onion, finely chopped
1 jalapeño pepper, finely chopped
1 teaspoon ground cumin
2 tablespoons extra-virgin olive oil, divided
2 teaspoons garam masala
2 cups low-fat plain yogurt
8 ounces paneer cheese, cut into 1/2-inch cubes
20 ounces frozen spinach, thawed and finely chopped

STEPS

1. Combine paneer with turmeric in a bowl until coated. Heat 1 tablespoon oil in a nonstick skillet over medium heat. Add the paneer and cook, until browned on both sides, about 6 minutes. Transfer to a plate.
2. Add the 1 tablespoon oil to the pan, onion, and jalapeño and cook, until golden brown, 8 minutes. Add garlic, ginger, cumin, and garam masala. Cook, stirring about 30 seconds. Add salt and spinach. Cook, stirring, about 3 minutes. Remove from the heat and stir in yogurt and paneer.

NUTRITION FACTS

Serving Size: 1 cup
Per Serving:

382 calories
protein 24.5g
carbohydrates 18.9g
fat 24g
cholesterol 64.1mg
sodium 641mg
fiber 4.6g
sugars 10.9g

Spinach Salad with Roasted Sweet Potatoes, White Beans & Basil

SALAD

PREPARATION
40 MIN

SERVES FOR
4 PEOPLE

INGREDIENTS

1/4 teaspoon salt, divided
1/3 cup chopped pecans, toasted
1/2 cup packed fresh basil leaves
1/2 teaspoon ground pepper, divided
1 sweet potato, peeled and diced
1 cup chopped red bell pepper
1 tablespoon finely chopped shallot
2 teaspoons whole-grain mustard
2 cups shredded cabbage
3 tablespoons cider vinegar
5 tablespoons extra-virgin olive oil, divided
10 cups baby spinach
15 ounce can low-sodium cannellini beans, rinsed

STEPS

1. Preheat oven to 400 degrees F.
2. Toss sweet potatoes, 1 tablespoon oil, 1/8 teaspoon salt, and 1/4 teaspoon pepper, in a bowl. Transfer to a rimmed baking sheet and roast, for 18 minutes. Let cool for 10 minutes.
3. Meanwhile, place basil, 1/4 cup oil, 1/4 teaspoon pepper, 1/8 teaspoon salt, shallot, mustard, and vinegar, in a food processor. Process until mostly smooth. Transfer to the bowl. Add bell pepper, pecans, spinach, beans, cabbage, and the cooled sweet potatoes. Toss to coat.

NUTRITION FACTS

Serving Size: 3 Cups
Per Serving:

415 calories
protein 11.8g
carbohydrates 44.3g
fat 23.6g
saturated fat 2.9g
sodium 564.5mg
fiber 14.7g
sugars 6.7g

Salmon & Fall Vegetables

FISH

PREPARATION
40 MIN

SERVES FOR
4 PEOPLE

INGREDIENTS

1/3 cup extra-virgin olive oil
1/2 teaspoon salt, divided
1/2 small head radicchio
1 pound fingerling potatoes
1 bunch broccolini, trimmed
1 tablespoon extra-virgin olive oil
1 pound salmon
1 small fennel bulb
1 tablespoon butter
2 medium heads Belgian endive
2 tablespoons sherry vinegar
2 cloves garlic, very thinly sliced
8 anchovy fillets
Bagna Cauda

NUTRITION FACTS

Serving Size: 3 Oz.Salmon, 2 Cups Vegetables & 2 Tbsp. Bagna Cauda Per Serving:

537 calories
protein 31.1g
carbohydrates 35.2g
fat 30.4g
cholesterol 67.4mg
sodium 704.6mg
fiber 7g

STEPS

1. Coat a large rimmed baking sheet with cooking spray.
2. Preheat oven to 425 degrees F.
3. Toss potatoes and broccolini in a bowl with 1/4 teaspoon salt, and 1 tablespoon oil. Transfer the potatoes to the prepared baking sheet. Roast the potatoes, for 15 minutes.
4. Push the potatoes to the edges of the baking sheet. Place salmon in the middle of the pan and season with the remaining 1/4 teaspoon salt. Arrange the broccolini around the salmon. Roast until the vegetables are tender and the salmon is just cooked for 10 minutes.
5. Meanwhile, to prepare bagna cauda: Heat oil and garlic in a saucepan over medium-low for about 2 minutes. Add anchovies and lightly crush until they flake apart, add butter and vinegar; cook over very low heat, for 2 minutes more.
6. Place the salmon, broccoli, potatoes, fennel, endive, and radicchio on a platter. Garnish with the reserved fennel fronds. Serve with the bagna cauda for dipping or drizzling.

Green Salad with Edamame & Beets

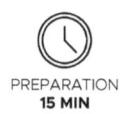

SALAD

PREPARATION
15 MIN

SERVES FOR
1 PEOPLE

INGREDIENTS

1/2 medium raw beet, peeled and shredded
1 tablespoon chopped fresh cilantro
1 cup shelled edamame, thawed
1 1/2 teaspoons red-wine vinegar
2 cups mixed salad greens
2 teaspoons extra-virgin olive oil
Freshly ground pepper to taste

STEPS

1. Arrange greens, edamame, and beet on a large plate. Whisk vinegar, cilantro, oil, salt, and pepper in a bowl. Drizzle over the salad.

NUTRITION FACTS

Serving Size: 4 Cups Salad
Per Serving:

325 calories
protein 18.5g
carbohydrates 25.5g
fat 15.7g
saturated fat 1.4g
sodium 682.2mg
fiber 11.6g
sugars 5.6g

Roasted Beet Hummus

HUMMUS

PREPARATION
10 MIN

SERVES FOR
10 PORTIONS

INGREDIENTS

1/4 cup extra-virgin olive oil
1/4 cup lemon juice
1/4 cup tahini
1/2 teaspoon salt
1 clove garlic
1 teaspoon ground cumin
8 ounces roasted beets, coarsely chopped and patted dry
15 ounce can no-salt-added chickpeas, rinsed

STEPS

1. Combine beets, chickpeas, tahini, garlic, cumin, salt, oil, and lemon juice in a food processor. Puree until very smooth, for 3 minutes.

NUTRITION FACTS

Serving Size: 1/4 Cup
Per Serving:

133 calories
protein 3.3g
carbohydrates 9.9g
fat 9.5g
saturated fat 1.3g
sodium 190.1mg
fiber 2.3g
sugars 2g

Peach, Raspberry & Watercress Salad with Five-Spice Bacon

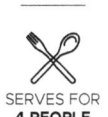

SALAD

PREPARATION
35 MIN

SERVES FOR
4 PEOPLE

INGREDIENTS

3/4 cup fresh raspberries
1/4 cup port
1/4 cup red wine
1/4 teaspoon Chinese five-spice powder
1/2 small head radicchio
1 tablespoon pure maple syrup
1 1/2 teaspoons Chinese five-spice powder
1 medium shallot, thinly sliced
1 teaspoon pure maple syrup
2 cloves garlic, peeled
2 tablespoons extra-virgin olive oil
2 tablespoons cider vinegar
3 firm ripe peaches
4 cups watercress, tough stems trimmed
8 ounces thick-cut bacon
Pinch of sea salt
Flaky sea salt for garnish
Five-Spice Bacon

NUTRITION FACTS

Serving Size: 2 Cups
Per Serving:

285 calories
protein 8.9g
carbohydrates 22.7g
fat 15.4g
cholesterol 20.6mg
sodium 364mg
fiber 3.3g
sugars 15.8g

STEPS

1. Cut bacon crosswise into 1/4-inch-thick strips. Heat a skillet over medium heat. Add the bacon and cook, for 5 minutes. Transfer to a paper-towel-lined plate. Pour the fat out of the pan.
2. Return the pan to high heat; add 1 tablespoon maple syrup, wine, port, garlic cloves, and 1 1/2 teaspoons of five-spice powder. Bring to a boil. Add the bacon and cook for 2 minutes, until the sauce is almost completely reduced, sticky, and coating the bacon. Remove from heat.
3. Mix shallot, vinegar, oil, syrup, five-spice powder, and salt in a bowl. Combine in raspberries, crushing slightly with the back of the spoon. Add peaches, radicchio, and watercress toss to coat. Serve the salad topped with glazed bacon. Garnish with flaky sea salt.

Turmeric Latte

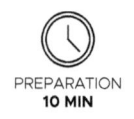

BEVERAGE

PREPARATION
10 MIN

SERVES FOR
1 PEOPLE

INGREDIENTS

1 pinch Ground cinnamon for garnish
1 teaspoon grated fresh ginger
1 cup unsweetened almond milk or coconut milk beverage
1 tablespoon grated fresh turmeric
2 teaspoons pure maple syrup
Pinch of ground pepper

STEPS

1. Combine maple syrup, milk, turmeric, pepper, and ginger in a blender.
2. Process on high until very smooth, about 1 minute.
3. Pour into a saucepan and heat over medium-high heat until steaming hot. Transfer to a mug. Garnish with a sprinkle of cinnamon.

NUTRITION FACTS

Serving Size: 1 Cup
Per Serving:

70 calories
protein 1.1g
carbohydrates 10.9g
fat 2.7g
sodium 172mg
fiber 1.1g
sugars 8.1g

Purple Fruit Salad

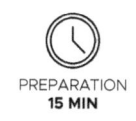

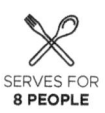

SALAD

PREPARATION
15 MIN

SERVES FOR
8 PEOPLE

INGREDIENTS

1 cup Lime Yogurt Fruit Salad Dressing
2 cups diced plums
2 tablespoons chopped purple basil
2 cups halved seedless black grapes
2 cups blueberries

STEPS

1. Combine blueberries, grapes, plums, and basil in a bowl. Serve with yogurt dressing.

NUTRITION FACTS

Serving Size: 3/4 Cup

56 calories
protein 0.7g
carbohydrates 14.4g
fat 0.2g
sodium 1.2mg
fiber 1.5g
sugars 11.4g

Beet & Goat Cheese Tartines

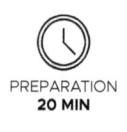

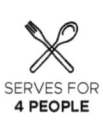

SIDE

PREPARATION
20 MIN

SERVES FOR
4 PEOPLE

INGREDIENTS

1/4 teaspoon salt
1 tablespoon extra-virgin olive oil, plus more for garnish
1 tablespoon white balsamic vinegar
2 tablespoons milk
4 small red beets
4 ounces soft goat cheese
4 slices crusty whole-grain bread, lightly toasted
Ground pepper to taste
Fresh thyme and/or flaky sea salt for garnish

STEPS

1. Bring 1 inch of water to a boil in a large saucepan fitted with a steamer basket. Add beets, cover, and steam until tender, for 15 minutes. Let stand on a clean cutting board until cool enough to handle. Rub off the skins with a paper towel. Cut the beets into slices. Transfer to a bowl and toss with oil, vinegar, salt, and pepper.
2. Stir goat cheese and milk in a bowl until smooth. Season with pepper. Spread about 2 tablespoons of the mixture on each piece of toast. Top with some of the beets and garnish with thyme and/or flaky salt.

NUTRITION FACTS

Serving Size: 1 Tartine
Per Serving:

225 calories
protein 10.6g
carbohydrates 21.2g
fat 11.1g
cholesterol 13.8mg
sodium 451.6mg
fiber 4.4g
sugars 8.3g

Spinach Salad

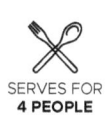

SALAD

PREPARATION
20 MIN

SERVES FOR
4 PEOPLE

INGREDIENTS

1/4 teaspoon minced garlic
1/4 teaspoon salt
1 large carrot, grated
1 medium red bell pepper
1 tablespoon ketchup
1 tablespoon reduced-sodium soy sauce
1 1/2 tablespoons finely grated fresh ginger
2 tablespoons distilled white vinegar
3 tablespoons minced onion
3 tablespoons peanut or canola oil
10 ounces fresh spinach
Freshly ground pepper, to taste

STEPS

1. Combine oil, ketchup, soy sauce, vinegar, onion, ginger, garlic, salt, and pepper in a blender. Process until combined.
2. Toss the carrot, bell pepper and spinach, with the dressing in a bowl until evenly coated.

NUTRITION FACTS

Serving Size: 1 1/2 Cups
Per Serving:

135 calories
protein 2.9g
carbohydrates 8.8g
fat 10.9g
saturated fat 1.9g
sodium 387.5mg
fiber 2.9g
sugars 3.6g

Turmeric-Ginger Tahini Dip

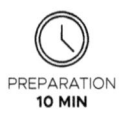

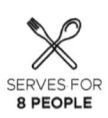

SAUCE

PREPARATION
10 MIN

SERVES FOR
8 PEOPLE

INGREDIENTS

1/4 cup rice vinegar
1/4 cup water
1/2 cup tahini
1/2 teaspoon salt
1 teaspoon grated garlic
1 tablespoon grated fresh ginger
2 teaspoons ground turmeric

STEPS

1. Whisk tahini, ginger, turmeric, garlic, salt, vinegar, and water, in a bowl until well combined.
2. Serve!

NUTRITION FACTS

**Serving Size: 2 Tbsp.
Per Serving:**

92 calories
protein 2.7g
carbohydrates 3.8g
fat 8g
saturated fat 1.1g
sodium 151.1mg
fiber 0.9g

Miso Soup Cup of Noodles with Shrimp & Green Tea Soba

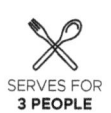

SOUP

PREPARATION
15 MIN

SERVES FOR
3 PEOPLE

INGREDIENTS

1 1/2 teaspoons dried wakame
1 1/2 cups cooked green tea soba noodles
3 teaspoons unseasoned rice vinegar
3 tablespoons thinly sliced scallions
3 inch square dried kombu
3 cups very hot water, divided
4 tablespoons white miso
5 ounces diagonally sliced snow peas
6 teaspoons mirin
9 ounces peeled cooked shrimp

STEPS

1. Add 2 tablespoon mirin, 2 miso teaspoons, and 1 teaspoon vinegar to each of three 1 1/2-pint canning jars. Layer 1/2 cup snow peas, 3 ounces shrimp, 1/2 cup noodles, and 1/2 teaspoon wakame, into each jar. Top each with 1 tablespoon scallions. Fit one piece of kombu between the ingredients of each jar. Cover and refrigerate for up to 3 days.
2. To prepare each jar: Add 1 cup of very hot water to the jar, cover and shake very well to dissolve the miso. Uncover and microwave for 3 minutes. Discard the kombu. Stir to make sure the miso is dissolved. Let stand a few minutes before eating.

NUTRITION FACTS

Serving Size: 2 Cups
Per Serving:

230 calories
protein 26.5g
carbohydrates 29.5g
fat 1g
cholesterol 160.7mg
sodium 788.9mg
fiber 2.3g
sugars 8.6g

Romaine Wedges with Sardines & Caramelized Onions

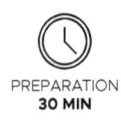

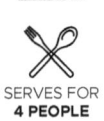

FISH

PREPARATION
30 MIN

SERVES FOR
4 PEOPLE

INGREDIENTS

1/8 teaspoon salt plus 1/2 teaspoon, divided
1/4 teaspoon freshly ground pepper
1/2 cup reduced-fat plain Greek yogurt
1 tablespoon canola oil
1 cup halved grape or cherry tomatoes
1 large sweet onion, sliced
2 tablespoons low-fat mayonnaise
2 tablespoons white-wine vinegar
2 tablespoons balsamic vinegar
2 hearts of romaine, halved lengthwise and cored
2 4-ounce cans of sardines with bones, packed in olive oil
4 teaspoons minced shallot

STEPS

1. Place oil, onion, and 1/8 teaspoon salt in a saucepan over medium heat. Cover and cook, for 15 minutes. Combine in balsamic vinegar and simmer, uncovered, for 2 minutes.
2. Whisk mayonnaise, yogurt, white wine vinegar, shallot, pepper, and the remaining 1/2 teaspoon salt in a bowl.
3. Divide romaine halves among 4 parts on a large platter. Spoon the dressing over the salads. Break sardines into two or three pieces each and divide among the romaine halves. Top with the caramelized onions and tomatoes.

NUTRITION FACTS

Serving Size: 1 "Wedge"
Per Serving:

202 calories
protein 14.4g
carbohydrates 13.5g
fat 10.4g
cholesterol 60.1mg
sodium 569.8mg
fiber 3.5g
sugars 6.6g

Orange, Anchovy & Olive Salad

SALAD

PREPARATION
15 MIN

SERVES FOR
4 PEOPLE

INGREDIENTS

1/8 teaspoon ground pepper, or more to taste
1 tablespoon fresh lemon juice
1 small red onion
2 teaspoons finely minced fennel fronds for garnish
3 tablespoons extra-virgin olive oil
4 small oranges
6 anchovy fillets
16 salt-cured black olives pitted

STEPS

1. Peel oranges cutting away all the white pith as well as the membrane that covers them on the outside. Working on a plate to help capture all the juice, slice the oranges into rounds thin.
2. Arrange the orange slices on a serving platter; conserve the juice. Distribute onion over the oranges, arrange olives over the top, and finally the anchovy fillets.
3. Pour the lemon juice and orange juice over the salad and drizzle with oil and pepper.
4. Let the salad stand at room temperature for about 30 minutes. Serve sprinkled with fennel fronds.

NUTRITION FACTS

Serving Size: 1 Cup
Per Serving:

202 calories
protein 3.1g
carbohydrates 14.6g
fat 15.2g
cholesterol 5.1mg
sodium 465.3mg
fiber 2.8g
sugars 9.8g

Spinach-Avocado Smoothie

SMOOTHIE

PREPARATION
5 MIN

SERVES FOR
1 PEOPLE

INGREDIENTS

1/4 avocado
1 teaspoon honey
1 cup nonfat plain yogurt
1 cup fresh spinach
1 frozen banana
2 tablespoons water

STEPS

1. Add spinach, banana, avocado, honey, yogurt, and water in a blender. Puree until smooth.

NUTRITION FACTS

Per Serving:

357 calories
protein 17.7g
carbohydrates 57.8g
fat 8.2g
cholesterol 4.9mg
sodium 237.mg
fiber 7.8g
sugars 39.3g

Roasted Root Veggies & Greens over Spiced Lentils

VEGGIES

PREPARATION
20 MIN

SERVES FOR
2 PEOPLE

INGREDIENTS

Vegetables
1/8 teaspoon ground pepper
1 teaspoon ground coriander
1 tablespoon extra-virgin olive oil
1 clove garlic, smashed
1 1/2 cups roasted root vegetables
2 cups chopped kale
2 tablespoons tahini
Pinch of salt
Fresh parsley for garnish

Lentils
1/4 teaspoon ground allspice
1/4 teaspoon salt
1/2 cup green lentils
1/2 teaspoon ground coriander
1/2 teaspoon ground cumin
1 teaspoon extra-virgin olive oil
1 teaspoon garlic powder
1 1/2 cups water
2 tablespoons lemon juice

STEPS

1. Combine water, lentils, 1/2 teaspoon coriander, cumin, allspice, garlic powder, 1/4 teaspoon salt, and sumac in a pot. Bring to a boil. Reduce heat to maintain a simmer, cover, and cook for 35 minutes. Drain. Stir in 1 teaspoon oil and lemon juice.
2. Meanwhile, heat oil in a skillet over medium heat. Add garlic and cook for 2 minutes. Add roasted root vegetables and cook, for 4 minutes. Add in kale and cook for 3 minutes. Stir in pepper salt, and coriander.
3. Serve the vegetables over the lentils, topped with tahini. Garnish with parsley.

NUTRITION FACTS

Per Serving:

453 calories
protein 18.1g
carbohydrates 49.7g
fat 22.4g
saturated fat 3g
sodium 346.1mg
fiber 13.9g

Tangerine & Roasted Beet Salad with Feta & Pistachios

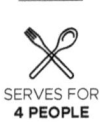

SALAD

PREPARATION
45 MIN

SERVES FOR
4 PEOPLE

INGREDIENTS

1/4 cup crumbled feta cheese
1/4 cup coarsely chopped toasted unsalted pistachios
1/4 teaspoon Dijon mustard
1/2 teaspoon salt, divided
1 tablespoon sherry vinegar
2 medium red beets
4 cups beet
6 teaspoons extra-virgin olive oil, divided
8 Pixie tangerines or clementines
Ground pepper to taste

STEPS

1. Preheat oven to 400 degrees F.
2. Rub the beets; wrap them in foil while still wet and place them in a pan. Cook for 1 hour. Let it cool for 25 minutes. Use a paper towel to scrub the peels. Trim the ends. Cut the beets into wedges. Rinse and drain the beets, set aside.
3. Grate 1/2 teaspoon of 1 mandarin zest. Slice the ends of all the fruit, then slice the peel and white pith, following the curve of the fruit. Cut the fruit into wedges and set aside. Combine the zest with vinegar, mustard, 1/4 teaspoon of salt and a generous grind of pepper in a bowl. Whisk in 4 teaspoons of oil. Add the beets and mix to coat; let it rest for 15 minutes.
4. Heat the remaining 2 teaspoons of oil in a non-stick pan over medium heat. Add the vegetables and the remaining 1/4 teaspoon of salt; cook, until wilted, for 3 minutes.
5. Divide the greens among 4 salad plates. Top with beets, fruit, feta, and pistachios. Drizzle with any remaining dressing.

NUTRITION FACTS

Serving Size: 1 Cup
Per Serving:

227 calories
protein 6g
carbohydrates 26g
dietary fiber 5g
fat 13g
cholesterol 8mg
sodium 325mg
sugars 18g

Green Tea-Peach Smoothie

SMOOTHIE

PREPARATION
10 MIN

SERVES FOR
1 PEOPLE

INGREDIENTS

3/4 cup unsweetened coconut milk beverage
1/4 cup fresh blueberries
1/4 cup silken tofu
1/2 cup diced avocado
1 teaspoon matcha tea powder
1 tablespoon coarsely chopped almonds
1 tablespoon unsweetened coconut flakes
1 teaspoon hemp seeds
1 cup frozen sliced peaches
2 teaspoons pure maple syrup

STEPS

1. Add peaches, tofu, avocado, coconut milk beverage, maple syrup, and matcha in a blender. Puree until smooth.
2. Pour the smoothie into a bowl and top with almonds, coconut, blueberries, and hemp seeds.

NUTRITION FACTS

Per Serving:

443 calories
protein 10.7g
carbohydrates 43.9g
fat 28.6g
sodium 35.6mg
fiber 13.1g
sugars 25.6g

Cranberry-Almond Granola Bars

BARS

PREPARATION
20 MIN

SERVES FOR
12 PEOPLE

INGREDIENTS

1/4 teaspoon salt
1/2 cup almonds, toasted and chopped
1/2 cup pecans, toasted and chopped
1/2 cup smooth almond butter
1 teaspoon vanilla extract
1 cup crispy brown rice cereal
1 cup dried cranberries
2/3 cup brown rice syrup
3 cups old-fashioned rolled oats

STEPS

1. Line oven baking pan with parchment paper, leaving extra parchment hanging over two sides. Lightly coat the parchment with cooking spray. Preheat oven to 325 degrees F.
2. Combine cranberries, almonds, pecans, oats, rice cereal, and salt in a bowl.
3. Add rice syrup, vanilla, and almond butter, in a microwave-safe bowl. Microwave for 30 seconds. Add to dry ingredients and stir until evenly combined. Transfer to the prepared pan and firmly press into with the back of a spatula.
4. For crunchie bars, bake until golden brown around the edge and somewhat firm in the middle, for 35 minutes.
5. Let cool in the pan for 10 minutes, then using the parchment to help you, lift out of the pan onto a cutting board. Cut into 24 bars, then let cool completely without separating the bars, about 30 minutes more. Once cool, separate into bars.

NUTRITION FACTS

Per Serving:

161 calories
protein 3.3g
carbohydrates 23.3g
fat 6.8g
saturated fat 0.7g
sodium 52.5mg
fiber 2.5g
sugars 10.7g

Blueberry Almond Chia Pudding

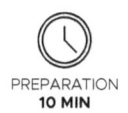

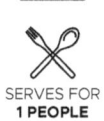

PUDDING

PREPARATION
10 MIN

SERVES FOR
1 PEOPLE

INGREDIENTS

1/8 teaspoon almond extract
1/2 cup fresh blueberries, divided
1/2 cup unsweetened almond milk
1 tablespoon toasted slivered almonds, divided
2 tablespoons chia seeds
2 teaspoons pure maple syrup

STEPS

1. Place together almond milk, chia, maple syrup, and almond extract in a bowl. Cover and refrigerate for at least 8 hours and up to 3 days.
2. When ready to serve, stir the pudding well. Spoon about half the pudding into a bowl and top with half the almonds and blueberries. Add the rest of the pudding and top with the almonds and blueberries remaining.

NUTRITION FACTS

Per Serving:

229 calories
protein 5.7g
carbohydrates 30.3g
fat 10.8g
saturated fat 0.9g
sodium 90.8mg
fiber 10.2g
sugars 15.8g

Citrus Salad with Ginger Yogurt

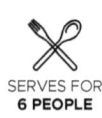

SALAD

PREPARATION
5 MIN

SERVES FOR
6 PEOPLE

INGREDIENTS

1/4 cup golden brown sugar
1/4 teaspoon ground cinnamon
1/2 cup dried cranberries
1 pink grapefruit, peeled
2 large tangerines or Minneolas, peeled
2 tablespoons honey
2/3 cup minced crystallized ginger
3 navel oranges
6 ounce greek yogurt
Dried cranberries

STEPS

1. Break grapefruit and tangerines into sections. Cut grapefruit sections into thirds; cut tangerine sections in half. Transfer grapefruit, tangerines, and all juices to a bowl. Using a sharp knife, cut all peel and white pith from oranges. Slice oranges into 1/4-inch-thick rounds then cut slices into quarters. Add oranges and all juices to the same bowl. Mix honey, cinnamon, and 1/2 cup dried cranberries cover, and refrigerate for at 1 hour. Mix ginger and yogurt in a bowl.
2. Add spoon yogurt atop fruit. Garnish with brown sugar and dried cranberries.

NUTRITION FACTS

Per Serving:

287 calories
fiber 3g
carbohydrates 60g
cholesterol 10mg
fat 4g
sodium 40mg
protein 7g

Red Bell Pepper, Spinach, and Goat Cheese Salad

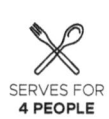

SALAD

PREPARATION
15 MIN

SERVES FOR
4 PEOPLE

INGREDIENTS

1/3 cup chopped red onion
3/4 cup crumbled soft fresh goat cheese
1 tablespoon chopped fresh oregano
1 1/2 large red bell peppers, diced
2 tablespoons extra-virgin olive oil
2 tablespoons fresh lemon juice
3 stalks diced celery
4 cups (packed) baby spinach leaves, coarsely chopped

STEPS

1. Add lemon juice, oil, and oregano to a bowl. Season to taste with salt and pepper. Add goat cheese, bell peppers, spinach, celery, and red onion to the dressing. Divide salad among 4 plates and serve.

NUTRITION FACTS

Per Serving:

155 calories
fat 11g
saturated fat 4g
cholesterol 10mg

Roasted Root Vegetables

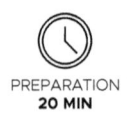

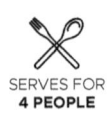

VEGGIES

PREPARATION
20 MIN

SERVES FOR
4 PEOPLE

INGREDIENTS

1/2-inch-thick slices
1 tablespoon extra-virgin olive oil
1 large sweet potato, peeled, cut in half lengthwise, and sliced
1 large or 2 medium turnips, peeled and cut into large chunks
2 medium beets red, peeled and cut into bite-size chunks
2 tablespoons maple syrup, blackstrap molasses
3 medium parsnips, peeled and cut into
4 medium carrots, peeled and cut into 1/2-inch-thick slices
Pinch each of ground cinnamon and nutmeg
Fresh rosemary leaves to taste
Salt and freshly ground pepper to taste

STEPS

1. Combine all the vegetables in a mixing bowl. Drizzle in the oil and maple syrup, then sprinkle in the cinnamon and nutmeg. Stir together.
2. Preheat the oven to 430 F.
3. Transfer the mixture to a lightly oiled roasting pan. Bake for 30 minutes, stirring every 5 minutes.
4. Toward the end of the cooking time, sprinkle on some fresh rosemary leaves. Season with salt and pepper; then transfer to a container. Serve immediately.

NUTRITION FACTS

Per Serving:

196 calories
fiber 8g
protein 3g
carbohydrates 40g
fat 4g
sodium 133mg

Brussels Sprouts and Carrots

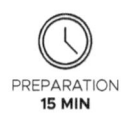

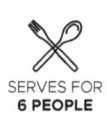

VEGGIES

PREPARATION
15 MIN

SERVES FOR
6 PEOPLE

INGREDIENTS

1/3 cup water
1 pound carrots, cut diagonally into 1/2-inch-thick pieces
1 pound Brussels sprouts, halved lengthwise
1 tablespoon cider vinegar
2 tablespoons chopped shallot
3 tablespoons unsalted butter, divided

STEPS

1. Cook shallot in 2 tablespoons butter in a skillet over medium heat, stirring occasionally, for 2 minutes. Add carrots, Brussels sprouts, 3/4 teaspoon salt, and 1/2 teaspoon pepper and cook, 4 minutes.
2. Add water and cover skillet, then cook over medium heat for 8 minutes. Stir in vinegar, remaining tablespoon butter, and salt and pepper to taste.

NUTRITION FACTS

Per Serving:

146 calories
protein 4g
carbohydrates 22g
fat 6g
saturated fat 4g
fiber 4g

Chilled Red Bell Pepper and Habanero Soup

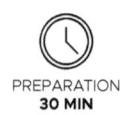

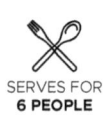

SOUP

PREPARATION
30 MIN

SERVES FOR
6 PEOPLE

INGREDIENTS

1/4 cup plus 2 tablespoons extra-virgin olive oil, divided
1 sweet onion, chopped
1 3/4 cups reduced-sodium chicken broth
2 pounds tomatoes
2 garlic cloves, chopped
4 medium red bell peppers
6 fresh habanero chiles, finely chopped, stems and seeds discarded

STEPS

1. Roast bell peppers on a broiler pan, turning with tongs until skins are blackened. Place to a bowl and cover with plastic wrap. Let stand 20 minutes. Peel, then halve lengthwise, discarding stems and seeds.
2. Cut a shallow X in the bottom of each tomato, then blanch tomatoes in simmering water for 30 seconds and transfer to an ice bath. Coarsely chop, reserving juices.
3. Cook onion, garlic, chiles, in 2 tablespoons oil, then add 1 teaspoon salt, and 1/4 teaspoon pepper saucepan over medium heat, for 8 minutes. Add tomatoes with juices, bell peppers, broth, and 1/4 teaspoon salt and simmer, covered for 5 minutes.
4. Purée soup in 3 batches in a blender, drizzling remaining 1/4 cup oil.
5. Leave to cool for 20 minutes and serve!

NUTRITION FACTS

Per Serving:

211 calories
protein 5g
carbohydrates 18g
fat 15g
cholesterol 0mg;
sodium 523mg
fiber 4g

Foil Packet Potatoes and Eggs

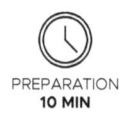

SIDE DISH

PREPARATION
10 MIN

SERVES FOR
4 PEOPLE

INGREDIENTS

1/4 tsp sea salt and black pepper each
1/2 tsp curry powder seasoning with turmeric
1/2 tsp smoked paprika
1 clove minced garlic
3 tbsp olive oil
4 cups of sliced golden
4 large eggs

STEPS

1. Slice your potatoes and toss them with olive oil and your seasonings.
2. Preheat oven to 400F.
3. Place about 1 cup of potatoes on grill sheet and bake at 400 F for 30 minutes, turning potatoes once, half way through cooking. While potatoes are baking, make your foil packets and place on a baking sheet.
4. Once potatoes are grilled, place 1 cup of cooked potatoes into each foil packet.
5. Crack an egg on top of each foil pack.
6. Place sheet pan back in the oven for 10 minutes.
7. Serve!

NUTRITION FACTS

Per Serving:

262 calories
protein 9.3g
carbohydrates 25.1g
fat 14.6g
cholesterol 186mg
sodium 243mg
fiber 2.8g
sugars 2.2g

Curried Chicken Salad with Spiced Chickpeas and Raita

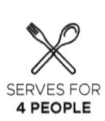

SALAD

PREPARATION
1 1/2 HOURS

SERVES FOR
4 PEOPLE

INGREDIENTS

For chickpeas:
1/4 teaspoon cayenne
1/2 teaspoon turmeric
1 tablespoon vegetable oil
1 teaspoon ground cumin
2 cups chickpeas, rinsed, drained, and dry
For curried chicken salad:
1 medium onion, chopped
1 tablespoon minced garlic
1 tablespoon minced peeled ginger
1 tablespoon curry powder
1 teaspoon ground cumin
1 cup plain yogurt
1 rotisserie chicken, meat coarsely shredded
1 cup red grapes, halved
2 tablespoons vegetable oil
2 medium tomatoes, chopped
2 tablespoons cilantro
For raita and topping:
1/2 cup sliced almonds, toasted
1 cup plain yogurt
1 seedless cucumber, peeled, cored, and chopped
2 tablespoons chopped mint
Equipment:
4 wide containers with lids

STEPS

1. Make chickpeas: Heat oil in a skillet over medium, then cook chickpeas, for 1 minute. Add turmeric, cayenne, cumin, and 1/4 teaspoon salt and cook, for 3 minutes.
2. Make the curried chicken salad: Cook garlic, onion, and ginger in oil in a skillet over low heat stirring, for 5 minutes. Add cumin, curry, and 1 1/2 teaspoon salt and cook, for 2 minutes. Add tomatoes and cook over medium heat, for 5 minutes. Transfer to a bowl and stir in chicken, yogurt, and cilantro.
3. Make raita: Stir together cucumber, mint, 1/2 teaspoon salt, and yogurt.
4. Assemble jars: Divide grapes among jars and layer curried chicken, raita, chickpeas, and almonds on top.

NUTRITION FACTS

Per Serving:

Calories: 635kcal
Carbohydrates: 49g
Protein: 45g
Fat: 30g
Saturated Fat: 6g
Fiber: 10g
Cholesterol: 109mg

Oat porridge with fruit

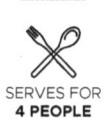

BREAKFAST

PREPARATION
30 MIN

SERVES FOR
4 PEOPLE

INGREDIENTS

Oats:
1 cup steel cut oats
3 cups water
pinch of salt
Topping:
fresh fruit berries
sliced almonds
hemp seeds
unsweetened kefir
a drizzle of maple syrup
coconut sugar

STEPS

1. Place a saucepan and over medium and add
2. the oats. Allow toasting, stirring frequently, for 2 minutes.
3. Add the water and bring it to a boil. Reduce the heat to a simmer, and let cook until the oats are tender.
4. Serve with seeds, berries and a splash of kefir.

NUTRITION FACTS

Varies on the type of fruit and oats you choose. **Check the nutrition label**

Dukkah Roasted

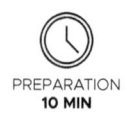

SALAD

PREPARATION
10 MIN

SERVES FOR
4 PEOPLE

INGREDIENTS

1/4 cup raw pumpkin seeds
1/4 cup olive
1 cup sliced peeled pearl onions
1 cup grape tomatoes
1 sprig of oregano leaves, to garnish
sliced lemon to garnish
1 tbsp or more dukkah
1 tsp minced garlic minced
1 cup chopped mixed greens (spinach, kale, shredded)
2 tsp lemon juice
2 mint leaves (chopped, to garnish)
2 cups sliced white button mushrooms
5 cups chopped cauliflower
pinch of black pepper
pinch of sea salt
Micro-greens or sprouts to garnish
crumbled feta or parmesan to serve
dried fruit to garnish

NUTRITION FACTS

Per Serving:

200 calories
protein 5g
carbohydrates 12g
fat 2g
cholesterol 1.6mg
sugars 5g

STEPS

1. Line a large sheet pan with parchment paper or grease.
2. Preheat oven to 400F.
3. In a bowl, place all your, mushroom, tomatoes, and onions diced/chopped cauliflower.
4. Add in 1/4 cup oil and then add in your dukkah spice mix, garlic, salt, pepper.
5. Mix in your chopped greens and toss.
6. Lay the chopped vegetables on the baking sheet and sprinkle the pumpkin seeds on top.
7. Season with pepper, salt, and fresh lemon juice.
8. Roast in the oven for 23 minutes.
9. Once cauliflower is golden brown, remove it from the oven and toss it in the pan.
10. Garnish with just a touch of fresh mint leaf, lemon slices, and a few leafs of fresh oregano.
11. Add extra olive, and in a few tablespoons of chopped dried fruit and crumbled feta.

Chickpea and Vegetable Coconut Curry

VEGGIES

PREPARATION
10 MIN

SERVES FOR
4 PEOPLE

INGREDIENTS

1/4 cup chopped fresh cilantro
1 teaspoon ground coriander
1 small head cauliflower, cut into bite-size florets
1 tablespoon extra-virgin olive oil
1 red onion, thinly sliced
1 lime, halved
1 red bell pepper, thinly sliced
1 tablespoon fresh ginger, minced
1 1/2 cups frozen peas
2 teaspoons chili powder
3 garlic cloves, minced
3 tablespoons red curry paste
4 scallions, thinly sliced
14-ounce coconut milk
28-ounce chickpeas
Salt and freshly ground black pepper

NUTRITION FACTS

Per Serving:

665 calories
protein 26g
carbohydrates 80g
fat 31g
sugars 17g

STEPS

1. In a saucepan, heat the olive oil over medium heat. Add the onion and bell pepper, for about 6 minutes. Add the garlic, ginger, and sauté for 1 minute.
2. Add the cauliflower and toss to combine. Stir in the chili powder, red curry paste, coriander, and cook until the mixture begins to caramelize for 1 minute.
3. Stir in the coconut milk and bring the mixture to a simmer over low heat. Cover the saucepan and continue cauliflower for 10 minutes.
4. Remove the lid and squeeze lime juice into the curry, stirring well. Add the peas, and chickpeas, season with salt and pepper, and bring the mixture back to a simmer. Garnish each portion with 1 tablespoon scallions, and 1 tablespoon cilantro.

Zucchini Taco

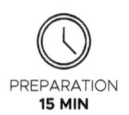

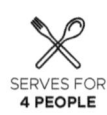

VEGGIES

PREPARATION
15 MIN

SERVES FOR
4 PEOPLE

INGREDIENTS

1/4 cup chopped green onion
1/3 cup shredded Cheddar cheese
1/2 cup water
1 teaspoon olive oil
1 cup fresh corn kernels
1 1/2 tablespoons taco seasoning mix
3 cups spiralized zucchini
3/4 pound lean ground beef
3/4 teaspoon salt
14-ounce black beans, rinsed and drained
14.5-ounce fire-roasted tomatoes with juices

STEPS

1. Heat oil in a skillet. Add beef; cook for 5 minutes, stirring to break up lumps. Increase heat to medium-high. Add taco seasoning and salt; cook, stirring often for 2 minutes more. Stir in beans, corn, tomatoes, and water; bring to a simmer, stirring. Simmer until slightly thickened, for 6 minutes.
2. Add in zucchini. Reduce heat low and cook, covered, for 2 minutes. Divide among 4 servings with cheese and green onion.

NUTRITION FACTS

Per Serving:

Calories 331
Fat 17.2g
Carbohydrate 21.5g
Cholesterol 69mg
Sodium 689mg
Protein 26.2g

Marinated Tomatoes and Mushrooms

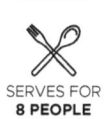

SIDE DISH

PREPARATION
25 MIN

SERVES FOR
8 PEOPLE

INGREDIENTS

1/4 cup balsamic vinegar
1/3 cup vegetable oil
1/2 cup chopped fresh basil
1/2 teaspoon salt
1/2 teaspoon ground black pepper
2 green onions, sliced
1 1/2 teaspoons white sugar
8 ounce package fresh mushrooms
12 ounces cherry tomatoes, halved

STEPS

1. Whisk together the vegetable oil, balsamic vinegar, sugar, salt, and pepper in a bowl. Add the onions, mushrooms, tomatoes, and basil. Toss until evenly coated. Cover and chill in the refrigerator for 4 hours. Stir before serving.

NUTRITION FACTS

Per Serving:

106 calories
protein 1.4g
carbohydrates 5.3g
fat 9.4g
sodium 153.3mg

Eggplant Caponata

SIDE DISH

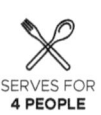

PREPARATION 30 MIN

SERVES FOR 4 PEOPLE

INGREDIENTS

1/4 cup olive oil, divided
1 teaspoon salt
1 eggplant, peeled and cut into 1/2-inch cubes
salt to taste
1 tablespoon tomato paste
1 teaspoon minced oregano
1 cup finely chopped celery
1 onion, finely chopped
1 clove garlic, minced
1 1/2 tablespoons drained capers
1 1/2 cups canned plum tomatoes, drained and coarsely chopped
2 tablespoons red wine vinegar
2 teaspoons white sugar
2 teaspoons minced fresh parsley
12 green olives, pitted and coarsely chopped
Ground black pepper to taste

NUTRITION FACTS

Per Serving:

54 calories
protein 0.9g
carbohydrates 4.9g
fat 3.9g
sodium 297mg

STEPS

1. Cook eggplant with salt and place in a colander set over a bowl. Let sit, about 35 minutes. Rinse and pat dry.
2. Heat 2 tablespoons olive oil in a skillet over medium heat. Add celery; cook, stirring often, about 3 minutes. Add garlic and onion, cook for 4 minutes. Transfer mixture to a bowl using a slotted spoon.
3. Heat the remaining 2 tablespoons olive oil in the skillet. Combine eggplant and cook, stirring constantly, for 7 minutes. Add in celery mixture, olives, capers, tomato paste, tomatoes, and oregano. Bring to a boil; reduce heat to low and cook for 16 minutes.
4. Season caponata with sugar, salt, and black pepper, and vinegar. Transfer to a serving bowl and garnish with parsley.

Indian Freezer Appetizer

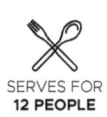

APPETIZER

PREPARATION
20 MIN

SERVES FOR
12 PEOPLE

INGREDIENTS

1/4 cup vinegar
1/4 cup olive oil
1 cup stuffed green olives, minced
1 cup black olives, minced
1 cup dill pickles, minced
1 red bell pepper, minced
1 green bell pepper, minced
1 cup marinated cocktail onions, cut in half
2 1/2 cups ketchup
5 ounce cans tuna, drained and flaked
14.5 ounce can green beans, drained
20 ounces canned mushrooms, drained and minced

STEPS

1. In a saucepan over medium heat, add the olive oil, pearl onions, canned mushrooms, green beans, green bell pepper, red bell pepper, green olives, black olives, dill pickles, tuna, ketchup, vinegar. Stirring, bring to a boil. Reduce heat and cook for 23 minutes.
2. Remove from heat. Allow cooling completely before transferring to freezer containers, leaving 1 inch of space in the containers. Store in the freezer.

NUTRITION FACTS

Per Serving:

22 calories
protein 1g
carbohydrates 2.4g
fat 1g
cholesterol 0.8mg
sodium 197.5mg

Artichoke Ricotta Flatbread

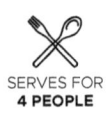

SIDE DISH

PREPARATION
10 MIN

SERVES FOR
4 PEOPLE

INGREDIENTS

LEMON VINAIGRETTE
1/3 cup olive oil
juice + zest of 1 lemon
2 teaspoons apple cider vinegar
Salt to taste

1/2 pound homemade at room temperature
1/2 cup fresh shaved parmesan cheese
1 tablespoon honey
1 tablespoon fresh chives chopped
1 1/2 cups fresh whole milk ricotta cheese
2 tablespoons fresh basil chopped
3 cups fresh arugula
8 ounces marinated artichokes drained
6 ounces fresh mortadella
Crushed red pepper flakes for sprinkling
Olive oil for drizzling

STEPS

1. Grease a large baking sheet with olive oil.
2. Preheat the oven to 460 degrees F.
3. On a lightly floured surface, roll the dough out until it is very thin. Transfer the dough to the prepared baking sheet and drizzle with olive oil, sprinkle lightly with salt and pepper. Place in the oven and bake for 10 minutes.
4. Meanwhile, stir together the ricotta, honey, a pinch of both salt, pepper, and basil. Remove the bread from the oven and garnish it with ricotta. Scatter on the artichokes and then sprinkle with crushed red pepper flakes. Add the torn mortadella. Garnish with fresh arugula and shaved parmesan. Just before serving drizzle with the lemon vinaigrette and chives.

NUTRITION FACTS

Per Serving:

551 calories

Lemon Chicken with Asparagus

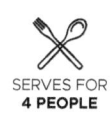

LUNCH

PREPARATION
10 MIN

SERVES FOR
4 PEOPLE

INGREDIENTS

1/4 cup flour
1/2 teaspoon salt, pepper to taste
1 lb. boneless skinless chicken breasts
1 teaspoon lemon pepper seasoning
2 tablespoons honey
2 tablespoons butter
2 tablespoons butter
2 lemons, sliced
2 cups chopped asparagus
Parsley for topping

NUTRITION FACTS

Per Serving:

232 calories
protein 27.5g
carbohydrates 10.4g
fat 9g
cholesterol 98mg
sodium 344mg
fiber 1.9g
sugars 1.4g

STEPS

1. Chicken: Cover the chicken breasts with plastic wrap and pound until each piece is 3/4 of an inch thick. Place salt and pepper the flour in a shallow dish and gently add each chicken breast in the dish to coat. Melt the butter in a large skillet over medium heat; add the chicken and saute for 3 minutes on each side, sprinkling each side with the lemon pepper directly in the pan.
2. Asparagus and Lemons: Add the chopped asparagus to the pan. Saute for a few minutes until bright green. Remove from the pan and set aside. Lay the lemon slices flat on the bottom of the pan and cook for a few minutes on each side without stirring so that they caramelize and pick up the browned bits left in the pan from the chicken and butter. Remove the lemons from the pan and set them aside.
3. Layer all the ingredients back into the dish– asparagus, chicken, and lemon slices on top and serve!

Garlic Shrimp

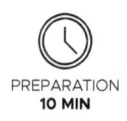

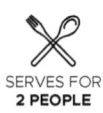

CRUSTACEANS

PREPARATION
10 MIN

SERVES FOR
2 PEOPLE

INGREDIENTS

3/4 pounds medium shrimp peeled & deveined
1 tablespoon olive oil
2 medium zucchini
4 cloves garlic minced
Salt & pepper to taste
Red pepper flakes
Juice and zest of 1 lemon
Chopped fresh parsley

STEPS

1. Cook the zucchini on the medium setting. Set aside.
2. Add the olive oil and lemon juice and zest to a skillet on low heat. Once the pan is warm, add the shrimp. Cook the shrimp for 2 minutes.
3. Add the red pepper flakes and garlic, cook for 1 minute, stirring.
4. Add the zucchini and stir constantly for 3 minutes until they're slightly cooked and warmed up.
5. Season with salt and pepper. Garnish with the chopped parsley.

NUTRITION FACTS

Per Serving:

276 calories
protein 38g
carbohydrates 9g
fat 10g
cholesterol 429mg
sodium 1339mg
fiber 2g
sugars 5g

Greek Chicken With Tomato, Olive, And Feta Topping

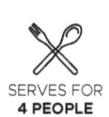

LUNCH

PREPARATION
20 MIN

SERVES FOR
4 PEOPLE

INGREDIENTS

1/3 cup sliced olives
1/2 cup olive oil
1/2 cup fresh-squeezed lemon juice
1/2 cup crumbled
1 cup cherry tomatoes
2 tsp. chopped fresh oregano
2 tsp. finely chopped fresh garlic
4 skinless chicken breasts, trimmed and scored on top
Feta cheese
Salt and fresh-ground black pepper to taste

NUTRITION FACTS

Per Serving:

552 calories
protein 41g
carbohydrates 3.1g
fat 38g
cholesterol 119mg
sodium 477mg
fiber 2g
sugars 8g

STEPS

1. Score the top of the chicken with small diagonal cuts that crisscross.
2. Mix together the olive oil, lemon juice, minced garlic, and oregano.
3. Remove 1/4 cup of that mixture and set aside for the garnish later.
4. Put scored chicken pieces into a baking dish for 2 hours.
5. Take the chicken out of the fridge and let it come to room temperature, and cut up the tomatoes and olives.
6. Mix together the cut crumbled feta, tomatoes, olives, and reserved marinade.
7. Heat 1 tsp additional olive oil in a frying pan.
8. Remove chicken from the marinade scored side down.
9. Cook for 8 min. Chicken should feel firm to the touch when it's done.
10. Season chicken with salt and fresh ground black pepper.
11. Arrange chicken on a platter and spoon tomato, olive, and feta topping, and serve!

Green Curry

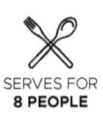

SIDE DISH

PREPARATION
15 MIN

SERVES FOR
8 PEOPLE

INGREDIENTS

2 sweet potatoes, peeled and cubed
3 cups broccoli florets
4 tablespoons green curry paste
12 ounces firm tofu
14 ounce of coconut milk
A swish of olive oil
Sprinkle of salt

STEPS

1. Tofu: Press the tofu with paper towels to remove water. Cut tofu into cubes, in a soup pot, heat the olive oil over medium heat, and add the tofu, sprinkle with salt, and pan-fry for 15 minutes. Remove and set aside.
2. Veggies: Add coconut milk, curry paste, and sweet potatoes, to the soup pot. Simmer for 10 minutes. Add broccoli and tofu. Simmer for 5 minutes until broccoli is bright green.
3. Serve!

NUTRITION FACTS

Per Serving:

305 calories
protein 7.5g
carbohydrates 14.5g
fat 26g
cholesterol 0mg
sodium 240mg
fiber 2.2g
sugars 2.6g

Roasted Fish with Vegetables

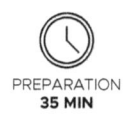

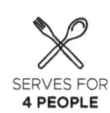

FISH

PREPARATION
35 MIN

SERVES FOR
4 PEOPLE

INGREDIENTS

1/4 cup pitted olives, halved
1/2 teaspoon sea salt
1/2 teaspoon freshly ground black pepper
1 Tbsp. dried oregano, crushed
1 lemon
1 pound fingerling potatoes, halved lengthwise
1 1/2 cups chopped fresh parsley
2 tablespoons olive oil
2 medium red, sweet peppers, cut into rings
2 cups cherry tomatoes
4 fresh skinless salmon fillets
5 garlic cloves, coarsely chopped

NUTRITION FACTS

Per Serving:

422 calories
protein 32.9g
carbohydrates 31.5g
fat 18g
cholesterol 78mg
sodium 593mg
fiber 5.7g
sugars 6.6g

STEPS

1. Preheat oven to 435 degrees F. Place potatoes in a bowl. Drizzle with a sprinkle with garlic and 1/8 tsp. of the salt and black pepper, and 1 Tbsp. of the olive oil. Transfer to a baking pan cover with foil. Roast 30 minutes.
2. Meanwhile, prepare salmon. Add in the same bowl, tomatoes, parsley, olives, oregano, sweet peppers, and 1/8 tsp. of the salt, black pepper, and with 1 Tbsp. of olive oil.
3. Rinse salmon and pat dry with the paper from the kitchen. Sprinkle with 1/4 tsp. salt and black pepper. Spoon sweet pepper mixture over potatoes and top with salmon. Roast, for 12 minutes more.
4. Remove zest from the lemon. Squeeze juice from lemon over salmon and vegetables. Garnish with zest.

Chicken Quinoa Fried Rice

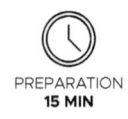

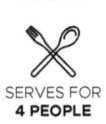

LUNCH

PREPARATION
15 MIN

SERVES FOR
4 PEOPLE

INGREDIENTS

1/2 cup diced red bell pepper
1/2 cup diced carrot
1/2 cup peas fresh
1 teaspoon toasted sesame oil
1 teaspoon peanut oil plus 2 tablespoons, divided
1 pound boneless, skinless chicken thighs, trimmed and cut pieces
2 large eggs, beaten
2 cups cold cooked quinoa
2 teaspoons grated fresh ginger
2 teaspoons minced garlic
3 tablespoons soy sauce
3 scallions, thinly sliced

STEPS

1. Heat 1 teaspoon oil in a skillet over high heat. Add eggs and cook, without stirring, until fully cooked on one side, about 35 seconds. Flip and cook until just cooked through, about 20 seconds. Transfer to a cutting board and cut into pieces.
2. Add 1 tablespoon oil to the pan along with garlic, scallions, and ginger cook, for 35 seconds. Add chicken and cook, stirring, for 2 minutes. Add bell pepper, carrot, and peas; cook, stirring, for 4 minutes. Transfer everything to a plate.
3. Add the remaining 1 tablespoon oil, add quinoa to the pan; and stir, for 2 minutes.
4. Add the chicken, vegetables, eggs to the pan, soy sauce, and stir. Garnish with sesame oil.
5. Serve!

NUTRITION FACTS

Per Serving:

425 calories
protein 31g
carbohydrates 27.4g
fat 20.5g
cholesterol 168mg
sodium 644mg

Lemon Chicken & Potatoes with Kale

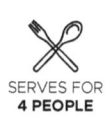

LUNCH

PREPARATION
30 MIN

SERVES FOR
4 PEOPLE

INGREDIENTS

1/2 cup chicken broth
1/2 teaspoon salt, divided
1/2 teaspoon ground pepper, divided
1 pound baby potatoes, halved lengthwise
1 tablespoon chopped fresh tarragon
1 large lemon, sliced
1 pound boneless, skinless chicken thighs, trimmed
3 tablespoons extra-virgin olive oil, divided
4 cloves garlic, minced
6 cups baby kale

STEPS

1. Preheat oven to 425 degrees F.
2. Heat 1 tablespoon oil in a skillet over medium heat. Sprinkle chicken with 1/4 teaspoon of pepper and salt. Cook, for 5 minutes and transfer to a plate.
3. Add the remaining 2 tablespoons oil, potatoes, and the remaining 1/4 teaspoon of each salt and pepper to the pan. Cook the potatoes cut-side down, for 4 minutes. Wisk broth, garlic, tarragon, and lemon. Return the chicken to the pan.
4. Transfer the pan to the oven. Roast until the chicken is cooked through and the potatoes are tender for about 17 minutes. Stir kale into the mixture and roast until it has wilted, for 5 minutes.
5. Serve!

NUTRITION FACTS

Per Serving:

374 calories
protein 24.7g
carbohydrates 25.6g
fat 19.3g
cholesterol 75.5mg
sodium 377.9mg
fiber 2.9g
sugars 1.8g

Chicken Kebabs with Mediterranean Couscous

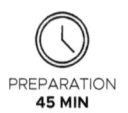

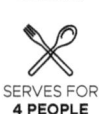

LUNCH

PREPARATION
45 MIN

SERVES FOR
4 PEOPLE

INGREDIENTS

Mediterranean Couscous
1/4 teaspoon salt
1/4 teaspoon black pepper
1/4 cup thinly sliced fresh basil leaves
1/4 cup snipped fresh parsley
1/3 cup plain fat-free Greek yogurt
1/2 cup couscous
1/2 cup snipped dried tomatoes
1/2 cup chopped cucumber
1/2 cup chopped red onion
1 teaspoon olive oil
1 cup water
1 tablespoon lemon juice
3/4 cup chopped red sweet pepper
Chicken Kabobs
1/4 teaspoon black pepper
1/4 cup lemon juice
1/3 cup dry white wine
1/2 teaspoon salt
1 pound skinless, boneless chicken breast halves, cut into strips
1 cup sliced fennel
2 teaspoons dried oregano, crushed
3 tablespoons canola oil
4 cloves garlic, minced
Lemon wedges

NUTRITION FACTS

Per Serving:
322 calories
protein 32g
carbohydrates 27.7g
fat 9.4g
cholesterol 82.8mg
sodium 360mg

STEPS

1. Prepare couscous: In a saucepan heat 1 teaspoon olive oil over medium heat. Add 1/2 cup couscous. Cook and stir for 5 minutes. Add 1 cup water. Bring to boiling. Simmer, covered, for 12 minutes, the liquid is absorbed, adding 1/2 cup snipped dried tomatoes the last 6 minutes. Stir in 1/2 cup each chopped cucumber and chopped red onion, 1/3 cup plain fat-free Greek yogurt, 3/4 cup chopped red sweet pepper, 1/4 cup each thinly sliced fresh basil leaves, and snipped fresh parsley, 1 tablespoon lemon juice, and 1/4 teaspoon each salt and pepper.

2. Prepare kabobs: Place chicken and sliced fennel in a plastic bag. For marinade, in a bowl combine the lemon juice, oil, white wine, garlic, salt, pepper, and oregano. Remove 1/4 cup of the marinade and set aside. Pour the remaining marinade over the chicken mixture. Marinate in the refrigerator for 2 hours. Meanwhile, 8 wooden skewers, soak e skewers in water for 40 minutes. Drain chicken, discarding marinade and fennel. Thread chicken, onto skewers. Grill chicken skewers, covered, over medium heat for 8 minutes, turning once. Remove from grill and brush with the reserved 1/4 cup marinade.

Greek Kale Salad with Quinoa & Chicken

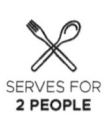

SALAD

PREPARATION
10 MIN

SERVES FOR
2 PEOPLE

INGREDIENTS

1/4 cup sliced jarred roasted red peppers
1/4 cup Greek salad dressing
1 ounce Crumbled feta cheese
1 cup cooked quinoa
1 1/2 cups shredded cooked chicken
4 cups chopped kale

STEPS

1. Place chicken, kale, roasted peppers, and quinoa in a bowl. Add dressing and toss. Top with feta.
2. Serve!

NUTRITION FACTS

Per Serving:

301 calories
protein 29.8g
carbohydrates 27g
fat 7.9g
cholesterol 42.2mg
sodium 378mg
fiber 3.7g
sugars 1.6g

Vegan Coconut Chickpea Curry

SIDE DISH

PREPARATION
20 MIN

SERVES FOR
4 PEOPLE

INGREDIENTS

1/2 cup vegetable broth
1 cup chopped onion
1 cup diced bell pepper
1 medium zucchini, halved and sliced
1 1/2 cups coconut curry simmer sauce
2 cups brown rice
2 teaspoons avocado oil or canola oil
4 cups baby spinach
15 ounce chickpeas, drained and rinsed

STEPS

1. Heat oil in a skillet over medium heat. Add onion, zucchini, pepper, and cook, stirring for 6 minutes.
2. Combine chickpeas, simmer sauce, and broth, and cook. Reduce heat to low and simmer for 6 minutes. Stir in spinach just before serving. Serve over rice.

NUTRITION FACTS

Per Serving:

471 calories
protein 10.9g
carbohydrates 65.8g
fat 18g
cholesterol 3.8mg
sodium 576.2mg
fiber 10.7g
sugars 12.3g

Sheet-Pan Chicken Fajita

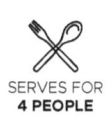

LUNCH

PREPARATION
20 MIN

SERVES FOR
4 PEOPLE

INGREDIENTS

1/4 teaspoon ground pepper
1/4 cup low-fat plain Greek yogurt
1/2 teaspoon garlic powder
1/2 teaspoon smoked paprika
1 medium yellow onion, sliced
1 medium red bell pepper, sliced
1 medium green bell pepper, sliced
1 tablespoon lime juice
1 1/4 pounds chicken tenders
2 teaspoons chili powder
2 teaspoons ground cumin
2 teaspoons water
2 tablespoons olive oil, divided
3/4 teaspoon salt, divided
4 cups chopped stemmed kale
15 ounce can no-salt-added black beans, rinsed

NUTRITION FACTS

Per Serving:

343 calories
protein 42.7g
carbohydrates 23.7g
fat 9.9g
cholesterol 70.9mg
sodium 605mg
fiber 8.2g
sugars 3.8g

STEPS

1. Preheat to 435 degrees F.
2. Place a rimmed baking sheet in the oven.
3. Combine 1/2 tsp. salt, garlic powder, paprika, and ground pepper chili powder, cumin, in a bowl. Transfer 1 tsp. of the spice mixture to a bowl and set aside. Whisk 1 Tbsp. oil into the remaining spice mixture in the bowl. Add onion, and red and green bell peppers, chicken, and toss.
4. Remove the pan from the oven and coat with cooking spray. Add the chicken mixture in an even layer on the pan. Roast for 17 minutes.
5. Meanwhile, combine black beans and kale with the 1 Tbsp. olive oil and 1/4 tsp. salt in a bowl.
6. Remove the pan from the oven. Stir the chicken and vegetables. Spread kale and beans evenly over the top. Roast for 7 minutes more.
7. Meanwhile, add lime juice, and yogurt, to the reserved spice mixture; stir to combine.
8. Divide the chicken and vegetable mixture among 4 portions. Garnish with the yogurt dressing and serve.

Cauliflower with Chickpeas

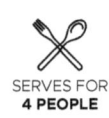

SIDE DISH

PREPARATION
20 MIN

SERVES FOR
4 PEOPLE

INGREDIENTS

1/4 cup water
1/4 teaspoon salt
1 tablespoon coconut
1 1/2 cups tikka masala sauce
2 tablespoons butter
4 cups cauliflower florets
15 ounce can chickpeas, rinsed
Fresh cilantro for garnish

STEPS

1. Heat oil in a skillet over medium heat. Add cauliflower and salt, cook, stirring occasionally, for 3 minutes. Add water; cover and cook for 5 minutes. Add sauce and chickpeas; cook, stirring occasionally, for 2 minutes. Remove from heat and stir in butter. Garnish with cilantro fresh.

NUTRITION FACTS

Per Serving:

268 calories
protein 7.8g
carbohydrates 26g
fat 15.9g
cholesterol 15.7mg
sodium 673.2mg
fiber 6.6g
sugars 4.1g

Plaice with Thai Coconut Curry Sauce

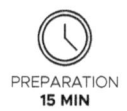

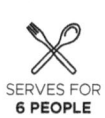

LUNCH

PREPARATION 15 MIN

SERVES FOR 6 PEOPLE

INGREDIENTS

1/4 teaspoon salt
1/4 cup thinly sliced fresh basil
1 cup coconut milk
1 cup green bell pepper
1 cup uncooked brown jasmine rice
1 1/2 cups water
1 1/2 pounds skinless flounder fillets
2 tablespoons canola oil
2 1/2 tablespoons Thai red curry paste
6 garlic cloves
14 ounces sweet potatoes peeled and cut into
14.5 ounce can no-salt-added diced tomatoes, undrained

NUTRITION FACTS

Per Serving:

332 calories
protein 18g
carbohydrates 40g
fat 10g
sodium 635mg
fiber 4g
sugars 5g

STEPS

1. The sweet potatoes in a sized microwavable bowl on High for 6 minutes, stopping to stir after 3 minutes.
2. Add the rice to a 6-quart slow cooker, and drizzle with the oil, stirring to coat evenly. Add the water, bell pepper, tomatoes, garlic, and sweet potatoes, stirring to combine. Cover and cook on high until the rice is tender and the liquid is absorbed, for about 3 hours.
3. Gently stir the coconut milk and curry paste into the rice mixture. Cover and cook on high until the liquid is absorbed for about 20 minutes. Place the fish on top of the rice mixture; sprinkle with the salt. Cover and cook on high, for 20 minutes. Serve the fish with the rice mixture, and garnish evenly with the basil.

Slow-Cooker Southwest Quinoa

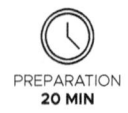

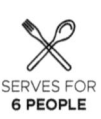

SOUP

PREPARATION
20 MIN

SERVES FOR
6 PEOPLE

INGREDIENTS

1/4 cup chopped fresh cilantro
1 cup fresh corn kernels
1 cup uncooked quinoa, rinsed
1 ripe avocado, cubed
1 tablespoon olive oil
1 teaspoon ground cumin
1 teaspoon chile powder
2 cups water
3 garlic cloves, minced
3/4 teaspoon salt
4 ounces Cheddar cheese blend, shredded
8 ounces yellow onion, chopped
8 ounces red bell pepper, chopped
15 ounce no-salt-added black beans, drained and rinsed
14.5 ounce can fire-roasted diced tomatoes

STEPS

1. Heat the oil in a skillet over medium. Add the onions and bell pepper; cook, for 6 minutes. Add the garlic, chile powder, and cumin, cook, stirring often, for 1 minute. Stir together the onion mixture, black beans, water, corn, tomatoes, quinoa, and salt in the slow cooker. Cover and cook on low until the quinoa is tender and the liquid is almost absorbed for 5 hours.
2. Add the cilantro to the slow cooker, stirring to combine. Sprinkle the cheese over the quinoa mixture; cover and let stand for 10 minutes. Divide the mixture among 6 portions.
3. Garnish with the avocado and serve!

NUTRITION FACTS

Per Serving:

364 calories
protein 15g
carbohydrates 44g
fat 16g
sodium 536mg
fiber 10g
sugars 7g

Italian Soup

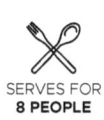

SOUP

PREPARATION
1 HR 30 MIN

SERVES FOR
8 PEOPLE

INGREDIENTS

Soup
1/2 cup freshly grated Romano cheese
1 tablespoon extra-virgin olive oil
1 cup chopped onion
1 cup chopped carrots
1 cup chopped celery
4 cups chopped cabbage
8 cups low-sodium chicken broth
8 cups coarsely chopped escarole
15 ounce white beans, rinsed
Sliced kale leaves
Meatballs
1/4 teaspoon salt
1/4 cup finely chopped fresh parsley
1/2 cup dry white wine
1/2 teaspoon crushed fennel seeds
1/2 teaspoon freshly ground pepper
1 pound ground turkey breast
1 cup fresh whole-wheat breadcrumbs
1 large egg, lightly beaten
1 tablespoon Worcestershire sauce
2 teaspoons extra-virgin olive oil
2 cloves garlic, minced

NUTRITION FACTS

Per Serving:

284 calories
protein 23g
carbohydrates 23.5g
fat 11.1g
cholesterol 60.1mg
sodium 522.5mg

STEPS

1. Soup: Heat 1 tablespoon oil in a soup pot over medium heat. Add onion, celery, carrots, and cook, stirring, for 8 minutes. Add cabbage and cook, stirring, for 6 minutes more. Stir in broth, escarole, beans, and meatballs, and any juice. Bring just to a boil, reduce heat to maintain a simmer and cook, stirring occasionally, and cook for 25 minutes. Garnish each portion with 1 tablespoon grated cheese.

2. Meatballs: Combine turkey, parsley, garlic, Worcestershire, fennel seeds, pepper, salt breadcrumbs, and egg, in a bowl. Refrigerate for 15 minutes to firm up. With damp hands, shape the mixture into 32 meatballs. Heat 2 teaspoons of oil in a nonstick skillet over medium heat. Add the meatballs and cook, turning occasionally, until browned on all sides, for 10 minutes. Remove from the heat and add wine, stirring to loosen any browned bits.

Chicken & Farro Herb Salad

LUNCH

PREPARATION
1 HR

SERVES FOR
6 PEOPLE

INGREDIENTS

Salad
1/4 cup chopped flat-leaf parsley
1/4 cup oil-cured black olives, sliced
1/4 cup fresh basil, very thinly sliced
1/4 cup fresh mint, very thinly sliced
1/4 teaspoon ground pepper
1/2 teaspoon salt
1/2 cup finely chopped red onion
1 fennel bulb, cored and chopped
1 cup diced carrot
1 cup chopped seeded English cucumber
1 cup farro
1 1/2 pounds boneless, skinless chicken breast, trimmed
2 cups arugula, tough stems removed, coarsely chopped
3 cups water
Red-Wine Vinaigrette
1/3 cup red-wine vinegar
1/2 teaspoon ground pepper
1/2 cup extra-virgin olive oil
1 small clove garlic, minced
1 1/2 tablespoons mustard
3/4 teaspoon salt

STEPS

1. Salad: Bring water to a boil in a saucepan. Add farro, reduce heat to low, cover and simmer for 25 minutes. Drain; transfer the farro to a bowl. Toss 1/3 cup of the vinaigrette with the warm farro; let stand until cool. Preheat a pan to high. Sprinkle chicken with pepper and salt. Oil the pan. Grill the chicken, for 15 minutes. Let cool for 6 minutes and slice. Stir carrot, onion, fennel, cucumber, parsley, basil, mint, and 1/3 cup vinaigrette into the farro. Just before serving, stir arugula into the farro mixture. Garnish the chicken and olives, with the remaining vinaigrette.
2. Vinaigrette: Combine the oil, vinegar, mustard, garlic, 3/4 teaspoon salt, and 1/2 teaspoon pepper in a bowl and whisk.

NUTRITION FACTS

Per Serving:

459 calories
protein 28.2g
carbohydrates 31.9g
fat 24g
cholesterol 62.7mg
sodium 512.6mg
fiber 5.3g
sugars 4.8g

Sheet-Pan Chicken & Vegetables

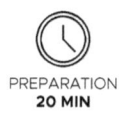

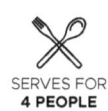

LUNCH

PREPARATION
20 MIN

SERVES FOR
4 PEOPLE

INGREDIENTS

1/4 teaspoon crushed red pepper
1/4 cup slivered almonds
1/2 teaspoon ground cumin
1/2 teaspoon salt, divided
1 small clove garlic, crushed
1 teaspoon paprika
1 teaspoon ground pepper, divided
2 tablespoons chopped fresh cilantro for garnish
2 large potatoes, cubed
4 tablespoons extra-virgin olive oil, divided
4 bone-in chicken thighs, skin removed, excess fat trimmed
4 cups broccoli florets
7 ounce jar roasted red peppers, rinsed

STEPS

1. Preheat oven to 435 degrees F.
2. Toss potatoes with 1 teaspoon oil, 1/4 teaspoon pepper, and 1/8 teaspoon salt in a bowl. Place on one side of a large rimmed baking sheet. Toss chicken with 1 tablespoon oil, 1/8 teaspoon salt, and 1/4 teaspoon pepper in the bowl. Place on the empty side of the baking sheet. Roast for 17 minutes.
3. Meanwhile, toss broccoli with 2 teaspoons oil, 1/8 teaspoon salt, and 1/4 teaspoon pepper, in a bowl. After the chicken and potatoes have roasted for 12 minutes, add the broccoli to the potato side of the baking sheet. Stir the vegetables together and continue roasting until the chicken is cooked through and the vegetables about 13 minutes more.
4. Meanwhile, combine roasted peppers, almonds, cumin, crushed red pepper, garlic, paprika, 2 tablespoons oil, 1/8 teaspoon salt, and 1/4 teaspoon pepper in a mini food processor. Process until fairly smooth.
5. Serve the chicken and vegetables with the roasted pepper sauce. Garnish with cilantro and serve.

NUTRITION FACTS

Per Serving:

500 calories
protein 33g
carbohydrates 29.5g
fat 26.6g
sodium 664.6mg
fiber 4.5g

Baked Salmon & Vegetables

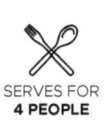

FISH

PREPARATION
25 MIN

SERVES FOR
4 PEOPLE

INGREDIENTS

1/2 teaspoon salt, divided
1 pound green beans, trimmed
1 large sweet potato, cubed
1 pound cremini mushrooms, cut pieces
1 1/2 teaspoons finely grated fresh ginger
1 1/4 pounds salmon, cut into 4 portions
2 tablespoons olive oil, divided
2 teaspoons rice vinegar
2 tablespoons chopped fresh chives
2 tablespoons honey
2 tablespoons reduced-sodium soy sauce
3 tablespoons tahini

STEPS

1. Place a rimmed baking sheet in the oven. Position one rack in the middle of the oven and another about 6 inches from the broiler. Preheat to 450 degrees F.
2. Combine mushrooms, sweet potato, 1 Tbsp. oil, and 1/4 tsp. salt in a bowl.
3. Remove the baking sheet from the oven. Spread the vegetable mixture in an even layer on the pan; roast for 25 minutes.
4. Meanwhile, toss green beans with the remaining 1 Tbsp. oil and 1/4 tsp. salt. Combine tahini, honey, soy sauce, and ginger in a bowl.
5. Remove the pan from the oven. Move the mushrooms and sweet potatoes to one side and place the green beans on the other side. Place salmon in the middle. Spread half of the tahini sauce on top of the salmon. Roast until the salmon flakes, for 10 minutes more. Turn the broiler to high; move the pan to the top rack and broil until the salmon is glazed about 4 minutes.
6. Stir vinegar into the remaining tahini sauce and drizzle it over the salmon and vegetables. Garnish with chives, and serve.

NUTRITION FACTS

Per Serving:

555 calories
protein 34.7g
carbohydrates 37g
fat 29g
cholesterol 78mg
sodium 718.4mg

Easy anti-inflammatory water

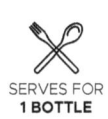

DRINK

PREPARATION
2 MIN

SERVES FOR
1 BOTTLE

INGREDIENTS

3 cups filtered water
1/4 tsp ground ginger
1/2 lemon juiced
1 Tbsp Pineapple juice without sugar

STEPS

1. Fill a bottle with filter water and add all other ingredients. shake the bottle for 30 seconds.
2. Drink throughout the day

Lemon Chicken Orzo Soup

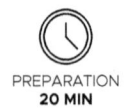

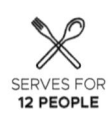

SOUP

PREPARATION
20 MIN

SERVES FOR
12 PEOPLE

INGREDIENTS

1/4 cup grated Parmesan cheese
1/2 teaspoon dried thyme
1/2 teaspoon dried oregano
1/2 cup fresh lemon juice
1 lemon, zested
1 lemon, sliced for garnish
1 onion, chopped
1 teaspoon olive oil
1 bay leaf
2 cloves garlic, minced
3 carrots, chopped
3 ribs celery, chopped
8 ounces orzo pasta
8 ounces cooked chicken breast, chopped
8 ounce baby spinach leaves
32 ounce fat-free, low-sodium chicken broth
Salt and ground black pepper to taste

STEPS

1. Bring a pot of lightly salted water to a boil. Cook orzo in the boiling water until partially cooked through but not yet soft, about 7 minutes; drain and rinse with cold water until cooled completely.
2. Heat olive oil in a pot over medium heat. Cook and stir carrots, celery, and onion in hot oil until the vegetables for 7 minutes. Add garlic; cook and stir until fragrant, about 1 minute. Season mixture with salt, black pepper, thyme, oregano, and bay leaf; continue cooking for another 45 seconds before pouring chicken broth into the pot.
3. Bring the broth to a boil. Partially cover the pot, reduce heat to low, and simmer until the vegetables about 12 minutes.
4. Stir lemon juice, lemon zest, and orzo, into the broth; add chicken. Cook until the chicken and orzo for 6 minutes. Add baby spinach; cook until the spinach wilts into the broth and the orzo is tender for 3 minutes. Ladle soup into bowls and serve!

NUTRITION FACTS

Per Serving:
Calories: 141.2kcal
Carbohydrates: 11.8g
Protein: 9.2g
Saturated Fat: 0.3g
Fiber: 2.3g

Charred Shrimp & Pesto

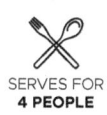

CRUSTACEANS

PREPARATION
25 MIN

SERVES FOR
4 PEOPLE

INGREDIENTS

1/4 teaspoon ground pepper
1/3 cup prepared pesto
1/2 teaspoon salt
1 tablespoon extra-virgin olive oil
1 cup halved cherry tomatoes
1 avocado, diced
1 pound deveined large shrimp patted dry
2 tablespoons balsamic vinegar
2 cups cooked quinoa
4 cups arugula

STEPS

1. Combine oil, vinegar, pesto, salt, and pepper in a bowl. Remove 4 tablespoons of the mixture to a bowl; set both bowls aside.
2. Heat a cast-iron skillet over medium heat. Add shrimp and cook, stirring, for 5 minutes. Remove to a plate.
3. Add arugula and quinoa to the bowl with the vinaigrette and toss. Divide the arugula mixture between 4 bowls. Top with avocado, tomatoes, and shrimp. Garnish each bowl with 1 tablespoon of the reserved pesto mixture.

NUTRITION FACTS

Per Serving:

429 calories
protein 30g
carbohydrates 29.2g
fat 22g
cholesterol 187.5mg
sodium 571.4mg

Turkey Meatballs with Linguine & Fresh Tomato Sauce

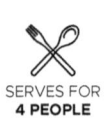

LUNCH

PREPARATION
25 MIN

SERVES FOR
4 PEOPLE

INGREDIENTS

1/4 teaspoon ground pepper
1/3 cup quick-cooking rolled oats
1/3 cup finely grated Parmesan cheese
1/2 teaspoon salt
1 teaspoon olive oil
1 egg, lightly beaten
1 1/4 pounds lean ground turkey
2 teaspoons dried Italian seasoning, crushed
3 cloves garlic, minced
8 ounces sliced fresh button mushrooms

STEPS

1. Line a shallow baking pan with foil; coat with cooking spray.
2. Preheat oven to 425 degrees F.
3. Heat oil in a medium skillet over heat. Place mushrooms; cook, stirring occasionally, for 10 minutes. Transfer the mushrooms to a food processor; process until finely chopped.
4. Combine oats, Parmesan, garlic, Italian seasoning, egg, salt, and pepper in a bowl. Add the mushrooms and turkey, and mix. On a cutting board, pat the meat mixture into a rectangle and cut it into 30 squares. Roll each square into a ball and place the balls in the pan. Bake until the meatballs for 16 minutes.
5. Divide the linguine and sauce between 4 plates. Garnish each serving with 6 meatballs.

NUTRITION FACTS

Per Serving:

467 calories
protein 36.3g
carbohydrates 49.2g
fat 16.1g
cholesterol 111mg
sodium 622mg
fiber 7.6g
sugars 8.8g

Chicken, Arugula & Butternut Squash Salad with Brussels Sprouts

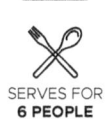

MEAT

PREPARATION
35 MIN

SERVES FOR
6 PEOPLE

INGREDIENTS

1/8 teaspoon ground pepper plus 1/4 teaspoon, divided
1/4 cup walnut oil or extra-virgin olive oil
1/2 cup very thinly sliced red onion
1 teaspoon extra-virgin olive oil
1 cup red grapes, halved
2 tablespoons white-wine vinegar
2 tablespoons finely chopped shallot
2 teaspoons mustard
2 3/4 cups pre cubed butternut squash
2 1/2 cups halved Brussels sprouts
3/4 teaspoon salt, divided
5 ounce baby arugula
10 ounces cubed cooked chicken

STEPS

1. Coat a rimmed baking sheet with cooking spray.
2. Preheat oven to 430 degrees F.
3. Toss 1 teaspoon olive oil, Brussels sprouts, squash, 1/4 teaspoon salt, and 1/8 teaspoon pepper in a
4. bowl. Arrange in a single layer on the prepared baking sheet. Roast, stirring once, cook for 23 minutes.
5. Combine chicken, grapes, onion, and arugula in the reserved bowl. Add the roasted vegetables and toss to combine.
6. Whisk vinegar, walnut oil, shallot, mustard, and the remaining 1/2 teaspoon salt and 1/4 teaspoon pepper in a bowl. Pour over the salad and toss to combine.

NUTRITION FACTS

Per Serving:

242calories
protein 17.4g
carbohydrates 17.5g
fat 12.1g
cholesterol 40.8mg
sodium 641.5mg
fiber 3.4g
sugars 7.1g

Roasted Salmon with Smoky Chickpeas & Greens

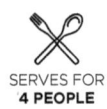

FISH

PREPARATION
40 MIN

SERVES FOR
4 PEOPLE

INGREDIENTS

1/4 cup mayonnaise
1/4 cup chopped fresh chives and/or dill
1/4 teaspoon garlic powder
1/4 cup water
1/3 cup buttermilk
1/2 teaspoon ground pepper, divided
1/2 teaspoon salt, divided, plus a pinch
1 tablespoon smoked paprika
2 tablespoons extra-virgin olive oil, divided
15 ounce no-salt-added chickpeas, rinsed
10 cups chopped kale
1 1/4 pounds wild salmon, cut into 4 portions

STEPS

1. Position racks in upper third and middle of oven; preheat to 450 degrees F.
2. Combine 1 tablespoon oil, 1/4 teaspoon salt, and paprika, in a bowl. Very thoroughly pat chickpeas dry, then toss with the paprika mixture. Spread on a rimmed baking sheet. Bake the chickpeas on the upper rack, stirring twice, cook for 27 minutes.
3. Meanwhile, mayonnaise, herbs, 1/4 teaspoon pepper, garlic powder, and puree buttermilk, in a blender until smooth. Set aside.
4. Heat the remaining 1 tablespoon oil in a skillet over medium heat. Add kale and cook, stirring occasionally, for 3 minutes. Add water and continue cooking about 4 minutes more. Remove from heat and stir in a pinch of salt.
5. Remove the chickpeas from the oven and push them to one side of the pan. Place salmon on the other side and season with the remaining 1/4 teaspoon each salt and pepper. Bake salmon for 7 minutes.
6. Drizzle the reserved dressing on the salmon, garnish with more herbs and serve with the kale and chickpeas.

NUTRITION FACTS

Per Serving:

447 calories
protein 37g
carbohydrates 23.4g
fat 21.8g
cholesterol 72.9mg
sodium 556.7mg
fiber 6.4g
sugars 2.2g

Jackfruit Barbacoa Burrito

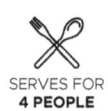

SIDE DISH

PREPARATION
20 MIN

SERVES FOR
4 PEOPLE

INGREDIENTS

1/2 teaspoon salt
1/2 teaspoon ground pepper
1/2 cup chopped fresh cilantro
1 cup unsalted canned black beans, rinsed
1 lime, quartered
1 cup chopped white onion
1 teaspoon chili powder
1 bay leaf
1 medium chile, stem and seeds removed
1 1/3 cups chopped plum tomatoes
1 1/2 cups unsalted vegetable broth
2 cups thinly sliced iceberg lettuce
2 tablespoons olive oil
3 cups hot cooked brown rice
6 garlic cloves, crushed
20 ounce green jackfruit in brine, rinsed and shredded

NUTRITION FACTS

Per Serving:

450 calories
protein 9.6g
carbohydrates 80.3g
fat 9.4g
sodium 755mg
fiber 22.1g
sugars 6.1g

STEPS

1. Heat oil in a saucepan over medium heat. Add garlic, onion, and chile; stir, and cook for 6 minutes. Add broth; increase heat to high and bring to a boil. Cover and reduce heat to medium. Cook until the chile is tender, about 10 minutes. Transfer the mixture to a blender. Remove the center piece of the blender lid; secure the lid on the blender. Place a clean towel over the opening and process until very smooth, about 40 seconds.
2. Return the chile sauce to the saucepan; add chili powder, salt, pepper, jackfruit, and bay leaf. Bring to a simmer over medium heat. Reduce heat to medium-low, partially cover, and cook for 8 minutes. Discard the bay leaf.
3. Place 3/4 cup rice in each of 4 shallow bowls. Top each with 3/4 cup jackfruit mixture, 1/2 cup lettuce, 1/3 cup tomatoes, 1/4 cup beans, and 2 tablespoons of cilantro. Serve with lime wedges.

Chicken, Quinoa & Sweet Potato Casserole

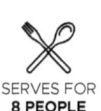

MEAT

PREPARATION
10 MIN

SERVES FOR
8 PEOPLE

INGREDIENTS

1/8 teaspoon cayenne pepper
1/4 cup fresh cilantro
1/3 cup dry white wine
1/2 teaspoon ground cinnamon
1/2 cup crumbled queso fresh
1/2 cup thinly sliced shallots
1 tablespoon canola oil
1 teaspoon salt
1 teaspoon ground cumin
1 1/2 cups multicolored quinoa
1 1/2 pounds boneless, skinless chicken thighs, trimmed
2 cups chopped seeded poblano chiles
2 tablespoons minced garlic
2 cups unsalted chicken broth
3 tablespoons water
4 cups cubed peeled sweet potatoes

NUTRITION FACTS

Per Serving:

349 calories
protein 22.9g
carbohydrates 38.7g
fat 10.5g
cholesterol 83.3mg
sodium 659.6mg
fiber 5.3g
sugars 5.7g

STEPS

1. Preheat oven to 425 degrees F.
2. Place sweet potatoes and water in a microwave-safe bowl. Cover with plastic wrap; pierce a few holes in the top with a fork. Microwave on High for 3 minutes.
3. Meanwhile, heat oil in a skillet over medium heat. Add chicken and cook until browned, for 6 minutes per side. Transfer the chicken to a clean cutting board and let stand 5 minutes. Cut into strips.
4. Add poblanos, shallots, and garlic to the pan and cook over medium stirring occasionally, for 3 minutes. Add quinoa, wine, salt, cumin, cinnamon, broth, and cayenne. Bring to a boil. Remove from heat and stir in the sweet potatoes and chicken.
5. Spoon the mixture into a broiler-proof baking dish. Cover with foil. Bake for 20 minutes.
6. Remove from oven; increase oven temperature to broil. Uncover the casserole and sprinkle with cheese. Broil 8 inches from the heat source until golden brown, about 6 minutes. Sprinkle with cilantro. Let cool for 5 minutes before serving.

Moroccan Baked Cod & Vegetables with Chermoula Sauce

FISH

PREPARATION
40 MIN

SERVES FOR
4 PEOPLE

INGREDIENTS

1/2 teaspoon salt
1 fillet cod, cut into 4 portions
1 teaspoon paprika
1 jalapeño pepper, seeded and sliced into rings
1 large russet potato, peeled and very thinly sliced
1 teaspoon ras el hanout spice blend
2 cups green bell peppers, cut into 1-inch pieces
2 green bell pepper, chopped
2 plum tomatoes, thinly sliced
2 lemons
2 tablespoons finely chopped fresh cilantro
2 tablespoons finely chopped fresh Italian parsley
3 tablespoons extra-virgin olive oil, divided
3 cloves garlic, minced

STEPS

1. Preheat oven to 450 degrees F.
2. Toss cauliflower, bell peppers, tomatoes, jalapeño, potato, 1 Tbsp. oil in a bowl. Transfer to a rimmed baking sheet. Roast, stirring every 10 minutes, until the vegetables are tender, about 20 minutes.
3. Meanwhile, zest and juice lemons. Mix the cilantro, parsley, garlic, paprika, lemon juice, and salt in a bowl. Combine in the remaining 2 Tbsp. oil.
4. Cut several slash marks into the top of each piece of fish. Place the fish, skin-side down, on the vegetables. Drizzle with the lemon juice mixture. Roast until the fish is cooked through and flakes easily, for 15 minutes. Sprinkle with lemon zest, and serve.

NUTRITION FACTS

Per Serving:

284 calories
protein 19.1g
carbohydrates 28.1g
fat 11.6g
cholesterol 44.6mg
sodium 609.7mg
fiber 4.8g
sugars 5.3g

Ratatouille

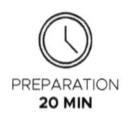

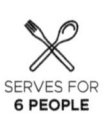

VEGGIES

PREPARATION
20 MIN

SERVES FOR
6 PEOPLE

INGREDIENTS

1/2 cup red wine
1 lb eggplant peeled, and cut into 1-inch pieces
1 tsp black pepper
1 tsp sweet paprika
1 tsp dried rosemary
1 tbsp sherry vinegar
1 medium-sized yellow onion finely chopped
1 red bell pepper stemmed, seeded, and cut into 1-inch pieces
1 green bell pepper stemmed, seeded, and cut into 1-inch pieces
2 lb vine ripe tomatoes chopped
2 zucchini halved lengthwise, then cut into 1/2 inch pieces
2 springs fresh thyme
3 tbsp chopped fresh basil
6 garlic cloves peeled, and minced
Salt
Extra virgin olive oil
To serve
Eggs over-easy fried in extra virgin olive oil
Crusty bread

STEPS

1. Place eggplant pieces in a colander and sprinkle with salt. Set aside for 35 minutes (the eggplant sweats out its bitterness.)
2. In a large heavy pot heat 2 tbsp extra virgin olive oil for 2 minutes. Add the onions. Cook about 4 minutes.
3. Add the green peppers and red peppers, cook for another 5 minutes.
4. Combine in garlic, zucchini, tomatoes, wine, eggplant, and fresh thyme springs.
5. Season with salt and add in the paprika, black pepper, and rosemary.
6. Bring to a boil for 7 minutes, stirring once or twice.
7. Turn the heat down and cook over low heat for 15 minutes.
8. Remove from the heat. Taste and combine with the sherry vinegar and a drizzle of extra virgin olive oil.
9. Sprinkle with fresh basil.
10. Place the ratatouille into dinner bowls add crusty bread on the side and a fried egg.
11. Serve.

NUTRITION FACTS

Per Serving:
Calories: 99kcal
Carbohydrates: 18.2g
Protein: 3.8g
Fat: 0.8g
Saturated Fat: 0.2g

Roasted Cauliflower

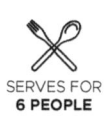

BREAKFAST

PREPARATION
15 MIN

SERVES FOR
6 PEOPLE

INGREDIENTS

1/4 cup toasted pine nuts
1 head cauliflower cored and divided into small florets
1 tsp harissa spice
2 tsp ground cumin
2 tbsp lemon juice
Salt and pepper
Handful fresh parsley for garnish
Extra virgin olive oil

STEPS

1. Preheat the oven to 450 F
2. On a baking sheet pour extra virgin olive oil and combine the cauliflower.
3. Add the cumin, harissa.
4. Season cauliflower with the spice mixture, black pepper, and a pinch of salt and toss to combine.
5. Roast for 25 minutes, occasionally rotating the baking sheet and turning cauliflower florets over, using a pair of tongs.
6. Remove from heat and carefully transfer roasted cauliflower to a serving dish.
7. Sprinkle with lemon juice, toasted nuts, and a little fresh parsley.
8. Serve

NUTRITION FACTS

Per Serving:

Calories: 27kcal
Carbohydrates: 5.2g
Protein: 2g
Fat: 0.4g
Saturated Fat: 0.1g
Fiber: 2g

Salmon Salad

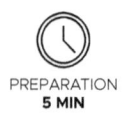

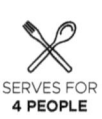

SALAD

PREPARATION
5 MIN

SERVES FOR
4 PEOPLE

INGREDIENTS

For Salmon
1 1/2 tsp Dried oregano
1 lb salmon fillet cut into 4 equal pieces
Salt and black pepper
For Salad
1 bell pepper, cored and sliced into rounds
1 English cucumber sliced into rounds
2 shallots sliced
8 oz chopped hearts of Romaine lettuce
10 oz cherry or grape tomatoes
pitted Kalamata olives
Quality Greek feta blocks
For the Lemon-Mint Vinaigrette
1/2 cup quality extra virgin olive oil
1/2 tsp sweet paprika
1 tsp dried oregano
2 large lemons
2 garlic cloves roughly chopped
25 fresh mint leaves no stems

NUTRITION FACTS

Per Serving:

Calories: 474.3kcal
Carbohydrates: 17.8g
Protein: 25.8g
Saturated Fat: 5g
Fiber: 5.5g

STEPS

1. Add olive oil, lemon juice, a pinch of salt, garlic, oregano, black pepper, paprika, and fresh mint in the bowl of a food processor fitted with a blade.
2. Blend until well-combined.
3. Set aside
4. Season the salmon on both sides with dried oregano, salt, and pepper.
5. Preheat the oven to 450 F.
6. Transfer the salmon to a lightly oiled sheet pan and brush the top of the salmon with extra virgin olive oil.
7. Bake the salmon in the heated oven for 10 minutes.
8. In a salad bowl, add the cucumbers, tomatoes, bell peppers, lettuce, shallots, and Kalamata olives.
9. Pour 1/2 of the vinaigrette over the salad.
10. Combine the feta cheese blocks on top. Remember to hold the remaining vinaigrette to dress the salmon.
11. Add to each salad bowl 1 salmon fillet and drizzle with vinaigrette.

Smoked Salmon

FISH

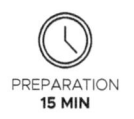

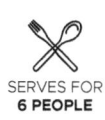

PREPARATION
15 MIN

SERVES FOR
6 PEOPLE

INGREDIENTS

1/4 cup assorted olives
1/3 cup marinated artichoke hearts
1 English cucumber, thinly sliced into rounds
1 bell pepper hinly sliced into rounds
1 vine-ripe tomato, thinly sliced into rounds
1 small red onion, thinly sliced into rounds
1 lemon, cut into wedges
3 oz Feta cheese, sliced into slabs
4 oz Cream cheese or Labneh
4 eggs, soft boiled
5 radishes, thinly sliced into rounds
12 oz smoked salmon
Salt
Red pepper flakes

STEPS

1. In a saucepan add water, eggs and boil over medium heat for 7 minutes.
2. Place the eggs in a bowl of iced water and let them sit for 3 minutes.
3. Peel the eggs, cut them in halves, and season with a pinch of red pepper flakes and salt.
4. Place in one-third of platter the labneh, in the other one-third, the feta cheese.
5. Arrange the bell peppers, tomatoes, salmon, cucumbers, radish, olives, onions, artichoke hearts, and lemon wedges around the cheese.
6. Drizzle a little more red pepper flakes.
7. Serve with pita chips if you like them.

NUTRITION FACTS

Per Serving:

Calories: 197.9kcal
Carbohydrates: 9.6g
Protein: 20.3g
Saturated Fat: 2.8g
Fiber: 2.1g

Eggplant Pizza Bites with Spinach and Mushrooms

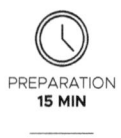

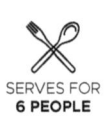

LUNCH

PREPARATION
15 MIN

SERVES FOR
6 PEOPLE

INGREDIENTS

1 eggplant, sliced into 1/2-inch rounds
1 cup homemade spaghetti sauce
2 cups fresh baby spinach
6 ounces sliced white mushrooms
10 oz fresh mozzarella
Salt
Extra virgin olive oil

STEPS

1. Heat the oven to 425 F.
2. Season the eggplant with salt on both sides.
3. In a pan with extra virgin olive oil place the eggplant slices in one single layer and brush the top of each eggplant slice with extra virgin olive oil. bake in the oven for 20 minutes.
4. In a medium skillet, heat about 1 tbsp extra virgin olive oil. Cook the mushrooms over medium heat for about 8 minutes, add in the spinach until it wilts. Season with a little bit of salt.
5. Take it out of the oven and top each eggplant slice with 1 slice of fresh mozzarella and 1 tablespoon of marinara sauce.
6. Return the sheet pan to the oven and broil for 2 minutes.
7. Remove the eggplant from the oven. Arrange the mushroom and spinach mixture over the eggplant slices.
8. Serve

NUTRITION FACTS

Per Serving:

Calories: 179.2kcal
Carbohydrates: 9g
Protein: 12.9g
Fat: 10.9g
Saturated Fat: 6.3g
Fiber: 3.4g

Lemon Roasted Broccoli

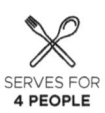

VEGGIES

PREPARATION
5 MIN

SERVES FOR
4 PEOPLE

INGREDIENTS

1 lemon zested and juiced
1 1/2 lb broccoli trimmed and cut into florets
1/2 to 1 teaspoon red pepper flakes
Extra-virgin olive oil
Salt
Feta cheese

STEPS

1. Put a rimmed sheet pan in the heated oven (to 450 F)
2. Trim the broccoli stems.
3. Add broccoli, 5 tablespoons of extra virgin olive oil, and a pinch of salt in a bowl.
4. Place the broccoli
5. into the sheet pan (use a pair of tongs).
6. Return the pan to the heated oven.
7. Roast for 7 minutes on one side.
8. Take the pan out and turn the broccoli over on the other side and cook for another 7 minutes.
9. Place the broccoli on a platter and sprinkle with red pepper flakes and salt.
10. Drizzle with a juice of one lemon, and a sprinkle of feta cheese.

NUTRITION FACTS

Per Serving:

Calories: 66.4kcal
Carbohydrates: 13.9g
Protein: 5.1g
Saturated Fat: 0.1g
Fiber: 5.3g

Speedy Salmon Patties

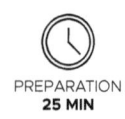

FISH

PREPARATION
25 MIN

SERVES FOR
3 PEOPLE

INGREDIENTS

1/8 teaspoon pepper
1/4 teaspoon salt
1/3 cup finely chopped onion
1/2 teaspoon Worcestershire sauce
1 large egg, beaten
1 can (14-3/4 ounces) salmon, drained, bones and skin removed
2 teaspoons butter
5 saltines, crushed

STEPS

1. In a large bowl, combine the first 6 ingredients. Crumble salmon over mixture and mix well. Shape into 6 patties.
2. In a large skillet over medium heat, fry patties in butter for 3-4 minutes on each side or until set and golden brown.

NUTRITION FACTS

Per Serving:

288 calories
protein 31g
carbohydrates 5g
fat 15g
cholesterol 139mg
sodium 1063mg

Minestrone

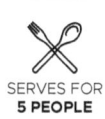

LUNCH

PREPARATION
10 MIN

SERVES FOR
5 PEOPLE

INGREDIENTS

1/4 cup extra virgin olive oil
1/2 tsp rosemary
1 tsp paprika
1 small yellow onion chopped
1 zucchini
1 cup green beans fresh or frozen, trimmed and cut into 1-inch pieces, if needed
1- inch Parmesan cheese rind optional
1 bay leaf
1 15- oz can crushed tomatoes
1 15- oz can kidney beans
2 cups already cooked small pasta such as ditalini
2 springs fresh thyme
2 carrots chopped
2 celery stalks diced
4 garlic cloves minced
6 cups broth vegetable or chicken broth
Salt and pepper
Large handful chopped parsley
Handful fresh basil leaves
Grated Parmesan cheese to serve

STEPS

1. In a Dutch oven, heat the extra virgin olive oil over medium heat for 2 minutes.
2. Combine carrots, onions, and celery cook tossing regularly for 6 minutes. Add the garlic and cook another minute.
3. Add the green beans and zucchini. Sprinkle with rosemary, paprika, and a pinch of salt and pepper.
4. Combine broth, crushed tomatoes, fresh thyme, bay leaf, and Parmesan rind.
5. Let simmer for 25 minutes.
6. Now add the kidney beans and cook for another 10 minutes.
7. Add the cooked pasta and simmer for 3 minutes.
8. Stir in the fresh basil and parsley.
9. Adjust salt and pepper to your liking.
10. Serve hot.

NUTRITION FACTS

Per Serving:

Calories: 211.9kcal
Carbohydrates: 26.7g
Protein: 6.8g
Saturated Fat: 1.5g
Fiber: 7.4g

Oven Roasted Tomatoes

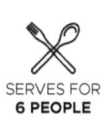

SIDE

PREPARATION
10 MIN

SERVES FOR
6 PEOPLE

INGREDIENTS

1/2 tsp dry chili pepper flakes
1 tsp sumac
2 lb Smaller Tomatoes, halved
2 garlic cloves, minced
2 tsp fresh thyme, stems removed
Extra virgin olive oil
Crumbled feta cheese
Salt and black pepper

STEPS

1. Preheat the oven to 450 degrees F.
2. Place the tomato halves in a bowl. Combine minced garlic, salt, pepper, fresh thyme, and spices. Drizzle with about 1/4 cup extra virgin olive.
3. Place the tomatoes on a baking sheet and Spread flesh side up.
4. Roast in your heated oven for 40 minutes.

NUTRITION FACTS

Per Serving:

Calories: 30.4 kcal
Carbohydrates: 5.6g
Protein: 1.4g
Fat: 0.5g
Saturated Fat: 0.1g
Fiber: 1.8g
Sugar: 4g

Florence White Bean Soup

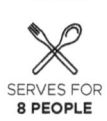

SOUP

PREPARATION 45 MIN

SERVES FOR 8 PEOPLE

INGREDIENTS

1 pound dried cannellini
1 tablespoon olive oil
1 cup diced carrots
1 cup diced celery
1 Parmesan rind
1 teaspoon salt
1 1/2 cups diced onion
2 dried bay leaves
2 tablespoons chopped fresh garlic
2 teaspoons minced fresh rosemary
3 tablespoons white-wine vinegar
4 cups low-sodium chicken broth
4 cups water
6 cups chopped fresh kale
15 ounce can no-salt-added diced tomatoes with basil, garlic & oregano, drained
Ground pepper to taste

STEPS

1. Rinse under cold water and transfer beans to a bowl. Combine 3 quarts of cold water, cover, and soak at room temperature for 12 hours. Drain the beans.
2. Heat oil in a pot over medium heat. Add celery, onion, and carrots.
3. Cook for 8 minutes. Stir in garlic; cook until fragrant.
4. Stir in broth, water, the soaked beans, bay leaves, and Parmesan rind. Increase heat to medium-high, bring to a boil, and cook for 5 minutes. Reduce heat to low, and simmer for 1 hour.
5. Add tomatoes, kale, tomatoes, and rosemary. Continue to cook for 30 minutes more.
6. Season with vinegar, salt, and pepper.

NUTRITION FACTS

Per Serving:

270 calories
protein 14.7g
carbohydrates 44g
dietary fiber 21.4g
sugars 6.6g
fat 3.1g
saturated fat 0.4g

Zucchini with Egg

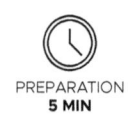

LUNCH

PREPARATION
5 MIN

SERVES FOR
2 PEOPLE

INGREDIENTS

1 teaspoon water, or as desired
1 1/2 tablespoons olive oil
2 large zucchini, cut into large chunks
salt and ground black pepper to taste
2 large eggs

STEPS

1. Heat oil in a skillet over medium-high heat; saute zucchini until tender, about 10 minutes. Season zucchini with salt and black pepper.
2. Beat eggs with a fork in a bowl; add water and beat until evenly combined. Pour eggs over zucchini; cook and stir until eggs are scrambled and no longer runny, about 5 minutes. Season zucchini and eggs with salt and black pepper.

NUTRITION FACTS

Per Serving:

213 calories
protein 10.2g
carbohydrates 11.2g
fat 15.7g
cholesterol 186mg
sodium 180mg

Creamy White Bean Soup

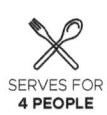

SOUP

PREPARATION
20 MIN

SERVES FOR
4 PEOPLE

INGREDIENTS

1/8 teaspoon dried thyme
1/4 teaspoon ground black pepper
1 tablespoon vegetable oil
1 onion, chopped
1 stalk celery, chopped
1 clove garlic, minced
1 bunch fresh spinach, rinsed and thinly sliced
1 tablespoon lemon juice
2 cups water
16 ounce cans white kidney beans, rinsed and drained
14 ounce can chicken broth

STEPS

1. Cook celery and onion in a saucepan with heat oil until tender. Add garlic, and cook for 30 seconds, continually stirring. Add in chicken broth, beans, thyme, pepper, and 2 cups water. Bring to a boil, reduce heat, and then simmer for 20 minutes.
2. Remove 2 cups of the bean and vegetable mixture from soup and set aside.
3. In blender at low speed, blend the remaining soup in small batches until smooth. Pour soup into the stockpot and stir in reserved beans.
4. Bring to a boil.
5. Stir in spinach and cook for 30 seconds. Stir in lemon juice and remove from heat and serve.

NUTRITION FACTS

Per Serving:

245 calories
protein 12g
carbohydrates 38.1g
fat 4.9g
cholesterol 2.4mg
sodium 1014.4mg